CNA

STUDY GUIDE EXAM TEST PREP

Pass the Certified Nursing Assistant Exam with Flying Colors!

Q&A | Tests | Extra Content

Blair Theo Ritter & Rory George

EXLUSIVE EXTRA CONTENTS FOR YOU IN THE LAST CHAPTER!

I have recently decided to give **gifts** to all our readers. Yes, I want to provide you with the assistance that will help you with your study you will receive:

Extra Content 1= **Audiobook**

Extra Content 2= Digital book **"Medical Terminology"**

Extra Content 3= Over **875** Flashcards (pdf and apkg. format *for Anki app or Anki droid*) divided into:

*__600 digital flashcards with picture__ of general medical terminology

*__275 digital flashcards__ covering a range of essential topics, including:

- Basic **anatomy** and **physiology** concepts
- Common **diseases** and **conditions**
- Common **medical abbreviations**
- Control and fall **prevention**
- Effective **communication skills** with patients and family
- **Laws** and **regulations** governing the CNA profession
- Pain **management** and wound care techniques
- **Procedures** and **techniques**
- Meal preparation and **nutrition skills**
- Safety **procedures** and **protocols**
- **Vital signs** and how to measure them

You can track your progress and conveniently and interactively memorize the most important terms and concepts! Learn with printable flashcards or interactive flashcards on your device with **Anki APP or AnkiDroid!**

TABLE OF CONTENTS

INTRODUCTION

The Certified Nursing Assistant (CNA) profession is essential to the healthcare system and provides advantages. In various healthcare settings, such as assisted living communities, nursing homes, and hospitals, certified nursing assistants (CNAs) are critical in providing patients with first care and assistance. They provide patients with daily care and emotional support in close collaboration with them. As a CNA, you can pursue a fulfilling career in healthcare, build your professional network, and dramatically enhance the lives of the individuals you seek.

CNAs often have their first interactions with patients, which emphasizes how important it is that they provide considerate care. One of a CNA's regular responsibilities is to assist patients with daily living tasks like cleaning, dressing, and grooming.
They also help with mobility, ensuring patients can safely move about their environment. CNAs also keep an eye on patients' health and let the nursing staff know about any changes. CNA is a rewarding career, even though it can be physically and emotionally demanding. One of the most rewarding aspects of becoming a CNA is building relationships with patients and their families. With a listening ear and a helpful hand, CNAs may significantly improve the comfort and well-being of the people they look after.

To become a CNA, you must complete a training program approved by the state and pass a certification exam. This process helps CNAs become more knowledgeable and proficient in their work, allowing them to provide the finest care possible for patients. A registered or licensed practical nurse oversees the training program, often combining classroom instruction with on-the-job clinical experience.

CNA training covers anatomy and physiology, nutrition, infection control, communication techniques, and basic nursing skills. By using this CNA Study Guide Exam Test Prep 2023-2024 to help you prepare for your certification exam, you can excel in your career as a CNA. In addition to covering the essential concepts and skills required to succeed as a CNA, the handbook offers strategies and recommendations to help you ace the test. This book also provides practice questions and resources to help you prepare for the test.

To sum up, becoming a certified nursing assistant is a challenging but very fulfilling vocation. Your hard work, dedication, and compassion will go a long way toward improving the quality of life for the patients you look after. You are choosing to change the healthcare business by following this career path. This CNA Study Guide Exam Test Prep 2023–2024 might be your reliable ally in becoming a compassionate and competent CNA.

WHAT IS A CNA

A medical professional with expertise in providing primary medical care to patients in various medical settings is known as a certified nursing assistant (CNA). CNAs help patients with multiple tasks that enhance their general health while working under the supervision of registered nurses (RNs) or licensed practical nurses (LPNs). Let's look at the CNA position and its significance in the healthcare system.
As a Certified Nursing Assistant (CNA), you will be directly involved in patient care, dealing with patients to ensure their comfort and basic needs are met. You will mostly be in charge of the following duties as a CNA:

- **Personal Care:** Assisting patients with their washing, dressing, and grooming needs is essential to a CNA's work. These tasks make this ongoing upkeep of patients' hygiene, decency, and self-worth possible.
- **Helping Patients Move:** Certified Nursing Assistants (CNAs) often help patients move throughout the hospital by dragging them from their beds to wheelchairs or other areas. It is imperative to employ appropriate protocols to mitigate the risk of injury to the CNA and the patient.

Feeding and nutrition: Getting the proper nutrients is essential for patients' health. CNAs can help feed patients, monitor how much food and beverages they consume, and report any problems to the nursing staff.

A CNA will regularly take a patient's temperature, respiration rate, blood pressure, and heart rate. Nurses and physicians need information like this to assess a patient's condition and choose the best course of action.

CNAs must have excellent communication skills because they constantly communicate with medical professionals and patients. CNAs are required to listen intently to patients' concerns and relay important information to nurses and physicians.

Support on an Emotional Level: CNAs provide emotional support for patients fighting their illness's psychological, physical, or emotional repercussions. CNAs profoundly positively affect patients' mental well-being by lending a sympathetic ear and a soothing presence.

In the healthcare sector, CNAs work in various locations, such as hospitals, assisted living institutions, nursing homes, and home healthcare agencies. Skilled CNAs are needed for this kind of care.

In hospitals, CNAs help doctors and nurses with patient care. In addition to helping patients with medical procedures and routine tasks to keep them safe and comfortable, they may supervise patients during their recovery. A certified nurse assistant (CNA) can provide patient care in many hospital departments, such as emergency rooms, intensive care units, and rehabilitation centers, for many patients, including the elderly and newborns.

Assisted living facilities and nursing homes are the two most common employment locations for CNAs. CNAs provide long-term care in these environments for residents unable to perform everyday duties independently. They work closely with patients and their families to create individualized treatment programs to guarantee that each patient's needs are met.

CNAs can also provide patients with essential care while they are at home in their own homes by working in home healthcare. In this scenario, CNAs assist patients with daily living activities, provide companionship, and monitor their health while working under the supervision of a home health nurse.

Regardless of the circumstance, the value of a CNA in the healthcare system cannot be overstated. CNAs significantly improve their patients' general health and well-being by providing appropriate care and emotional support. They also contribute significantly to the team by working with other medical professionals to provide careful and comprehensive oversight.

A Certified Nursing Assistant (CNA) is responsible for providing patients with essential care in various healthcare settings, making them an integral healthcare team member. CNAs assist patients with daily duties, monitor vital signs, and offer emotional support to ensure they receive the attention and care they need as they rehabilitate. Furthermore, CNAs collaborate with physicians, nurses, and other healthcare professionals to provide superior, patient-focused care.

The work of a CNA is multifaceted and demands a unique blend of people skills, emotional toughness, and professional knowledge. CNAs work with people of diverse ages and health conditions, so they need to be sensitive, adaptable, and detail-oriented. They must also be excellent communicators to inform the other healthcare team members about the patient's needs and concerns.

In addition to these fundamental traits, a successful CNA is committed to professional development and lifetime learning. The healthcare industry is ever-evolving. CNAS must be current on industry standards, best practices, and new products to perform their duties efficiently and knowledgeably.

It's also crucial to recognize the wealth of opportunities for professional advancement that the CNA occupation offers. With additional training and education, CNAs might specialize in a particular area of healthcare, such as pediatrics, geriatrics, or mental health. If they fulfill the educational and licensing requirements, they can pursue advanced nursing roles such as registered nurse (RN) or licensed practical nurse (LPN).

A Certified Nursing Assistant has a significant and rewarding role in healthcare. CNAs have a unique opportunity to enhance patients' lives while fostering a sense of camaraderie and teamwork among healthcare team members. The comprehension, expertise, and individual growth of CNAs

TRAINING AND CERTIFICATION REQUIREMENTS

To begin a job as a nurse assistant, one must complete training and certification as a Certified Nursing Assistant (CNA). This section goes to great length about these requirements, reviewing things like educational background, training courses, state certification examinations, and further professional development. When starting a career as a CNA, better understanding these prerequisites will increase your chances of success.

Obtaining a GED or high school diploma is the prerequisite for working as a CNA. Your employment opportunities can be improved, and the groundwork for future professional advancement can be laid with a GED or certificate.

After graduating high school, you must finish a state-approved program to become a CNA. Healthcare facilities, vocational schools, and community colleges offer these programs. This program may last for a maximum of 12 weeks, depending on how long it is.

CNA training programs combine didactic instruction with practical clinical experience. Essential topics covered in class include anatomy and physiology, infection prevention, medical terminology, and basic nursing skills. Under the guidance of an RN or LPN, clinical practice allows students to apply their knowledge in practical settings.

State Certification Exam: It's time to take the state certification exam after finishing a CNA training program approved by the state. This exam has **two** parts: a skills evaluation and a written (or oral) test. Multiple-choice questions on patient care, infection control, and communication are included in the written exam. As part of the skills exam, candidates must do real-world tasks for an assessor to see, such as taking a patient's vital signs or helping them with personal hygiene.

You must get good scores on the written and skills exams to pass the state certification exam. Upon passing the exam, you will become a Certified Nursing Assistant and have your name legally placed in the nursing aide register in your state.

Background Check and Additional Requirements: You may also need to pass a tuberculosis test, a drug test, and a background check in addition to completing the state certification exam. These requirements guarantee that CNAs uphold the greatest professionalism and can give their patients safe, morally responsible care.

Continuing Education and Licence Renewal: CNAS must be current on state laws, industry advancements, and best practices. You must finish a certain number of continuing education units (CEUs) and renew your license regularly with your state's regulations to get your certification.

A few options for continuing education are conferences, seminars, workshops, and online courses. Participating in these events can expand your network, strengthen your professional network, and learn new information. As a CNA, you have access to training and ongoing education. You can increase your income and take on more responsibilities by enrolling in an LPN or RN program. It might also be feasible to specialize in a particular field of medicine, such as pediatrics, mental health, or geriatrics, through further education and certification programs.

To become a Certified Nursing Assistant, you must complete additional background checks, pass the state certification exam, have a high school diploma or GED, and enroll in a state-approved CNA training program. To maintain their licenses, CNAs must also renew them and fulfill continuing education requirements.

Typical Responsibilities and Challenges of a CNA

Being a Certified Nursing Assistant (CNA) entails several duties and difficulties. This section describes the regular tasks performed by CNAs and potential daily obstacles. Knowledge of these facets of the work will help you better position yourself for a prosperous career in this fulfilling industry.

- **Providing Personal Care:** Assisting patients with personal care duties like washing, dressing, grooming, and using the restroom is one of a CNA's primary duties. These responsibilities safeguard patients' hygiene and dignity while advancing their general well-being. Personal care can be a delicate and private process for patients, so CNAs need to be kind and considerate when giving it.
- **Helping with Mobility:** CNAs frequently assist patients with trouble moving around a medical institution. This assistance may be pushing them while they walk or transporting them between beds and wheelchairs. CNAs must be proficient in safe lifting and transfer practices to reduce the risk of injury to themselves and their patients.
- **Monitoring and Recording Patient Care:** CNAs are essential in keeping track of patients' health conditions and monitoring them. This entails monitoring vital signs, informing nursing personnel of patient health changes, and recording pertinent data in patients' charts. CNAs must be meticulous and communicate on time to perform their jobs.
- **Helping with Meals and Nutrition:** A CNA's primary duty is guaranteeing patients enough nourishment. In addition to recording food and hydration consumption and reporting any problems or changes in eating patterns to the nursing team, they may assist patients with eating. CNAs ought to be aware of dietary limitations and considerate of the needs and preferences of their patients.

Providing Emotional Support: For patients experiencing emotional, mental, or physical difficulties due to their medical problems, CNAs are frequently their primary source of support; CNAs substantially impact their patients' emotional health by listening sympathetically and being comforting.

Challenges CNAs May Encounter

- **Physical Demands:** Because CNAs must spend a lot of time on their feet, lift and move patients, and complete repetitive duties, the job can be physically taxing. To reduce the risk of injury and burnout, CNAs should prioritize taking care of themselves, maintaining good body mechanics, and taking breaks when needed.
- **Emotional Stress:** CNAs may experience emotional exhaustion when caring for patients who are ill, in pain, or have lost a loved one. Creating good coping strategies, asking coworkers for assistance, and utilizing resources like counseling or support groups can all help CNAs deal with the emotional demands of their jobs.
- **Time management:** CNAs must possess strong time management and prioritization skills to manage their many obligations effectively and attend to the various requirements of their patients. CNAs can manage their hectic workdays more effectively by developing organizational skills and knowing when to assign responsibilities.
- **Complicated Patients or Families:** CNAs may deal with complex patients or families that are irrational, demanding, or even violent. In these circumstances, remaining professional and using good communication techniques can assist in easing tensions and guarantee the patient receives the best care possible.
- **Ethical Dilemmas:** CNAs occasionally encounter moral conundrums, such as when patients' desires contradict the recommended care plan or when they observe unethical behavior by coworkers. It might be challenging to navigate these situations, but CNAs can make wise decisions by studying pertinent ethical rules or asking supervisors for advice.

In summary, a CNA must overcome various obstacles while performing multiple duties, including emotional support and personal care. Knowing these things and acquiring the required abilities and coping mechanisms will help you succeed as a CNA.

ESSENTIAL SKILLS

Becoming a successful Certified Nursing Assistant (CNA) is necessary to gain proficiency in several crucial areas. The essential skills CNAs require to succeed in their employment and deliver top-notch patient care will be covered in this chapter. These abilities will help you stand out and improve your professional effectiveness.

- **Communication Skills:** CNAs must communicate effectively to provide important information to patients, their families, and the healthcare team. To make sure their message is understood, CNAs need to be able to talk effectively, listen intently, and use nonverbal clues. Strong communication abilities are also essential for CNAs to build relationships with patients and inspire confidence in the care they deliver.

- **Observation and Documentation:** CNAs play a vital role in keeping track of patient's health and recording pertinent data. They have to monitor the patient's vital signs, notice any changes in their condition, and precisely report what they see. To guarantee that the medical team has the knowledge necessary to make educated decisions on patient care, meticulous documentation and attention to detail are crucial.

- **Time management and organization:** CNAs face everyday challenges in juggling various jobs and duties. To guarantee that every patient receives the proper treatment, they must be adept in time management, task prioritization, and organizational skills. CNAs must multitask, adjust to changing circumstances, and stay focused under duress.

- **Patient Care Skills:** Certified Nurse Assistants (CNAs) must be skilled in various patient care procedures, including cleaning, dressing, grooming, and helping with mobility. Physical prowess and empathy for patients' needs and preferences are prerequisites for these roles. CNAs can improve patients' well-being and dignity by providing individualized, empathetic care by learning these care skills.

- **Safety and Infection Control:** To safeguard themselves, their patients, and their coworkers, CNAs need to be aware of safety precautions and infection control practices. This entails using personal protection equipment (PPE), being aware of good hand hygiene, and following the facility's cleaning and disinfection protocols. In addition to avoiding workplace mishaps, CNAs should know how to handle and dispose of hazardous chemicals securely.

- **Basic Medical Knowledge:** Certified Nursing Assistants (CNAs) must possess a firm grasp of fundamental medical principles, including anatomy, physiology, and medical terminology. With this understanding, they are better equipped to interact with other medical experts and understand the care plans created by the healthcare team.

- **Cultural Competence:** Since CNAs frequently care for patients from various backgrounds, they must possess this ability. This entails recognizing cultural variances, honoring patients' customs and beliefs, and modifying care to suit each patient's individual needs. CNAs that exhibit cultural competency can create a warm, inviting atmosphere that promotes favorable patient outcomes.

- **Compassion & Empathy:** Compassion and empathy are the foundation of high-quality patient care. CNAs need to be able to put themselves in their patients' positions, comprehend their needs and feelings, and offer consolation and assurance when things get tough. Being compassionate and empathic helps patients and also makes CNAs happier in their jobs.

- Another crucial duty of CNAs is collaborating with physicians, nurses, therapists, and other medical specialists as part of a multidisciplinary team. For a workplace to be productive, they must share knowledge and communicate clearly. CNAs need to have good collaborative skills to give their patients the best care possible and contribute to the overall success of their institutions.

- **Upholding ethical and professional standards:** CNAs should act professionally at all times. Patient privacy must be maintained, individual liberty and rights must be supported, and all actions must be morally and responsibly undertaken. Maintaining these standards is essential for CNAS to build confidence with its patients and colleagues and a strong reputation in the healthcare sector.

- **Handling stress and burnout:** If stress and burnout are not effectively managed, a CNA's hard job may lead to anxiety and burnout. Coping strategies will enable CNAs to handle the daily psychological and physical difficulties they encounter. Taking care of oneself, asking for assistance from coworkers, and upholding a healthy work-life balance are all necessary for a successful work-life balance. CNAs that possess resilience are better able to handle the highs and lows of their work and deliver high-quality care.

- **Adaptability and Problem-Solving:** In the always-evolving healthcare environment, CNAs need to be able to think on their own and be flexible. They must be equipped to handle unforeseen circumstances, such as staffing shortages or emergencies, and develop strategies to get past roadblocks. CNAs that possess problem-solving abilities are better able to offer care and have more professional progress and happiness.

In conclusion, to succeed in their jobs and give their patients the best care possible, CNAs need to become proficient in various critical abilities. You may improve your professional competence, handle the demands of your work more skillfully, and ultimately have a good impact on the lives of the patients you serve if you concentrate on honing these skills.

Prioritizing essential skills such as communication, empathy, teamwork, and adaptability can help you succeed as a CNA and foster a caring and compassionate healthcare environment for everyone.

ASSISTING PATIENTS WITH DAILY ACTIVITIES

Helping patients with everyday tasks like eating, moving about, and taking care of themselves is one of the primary responsibilities of a Certified Nursing Assistant (CNA). By becoming aware of the best ways to support patients' independence, dignity, and well-being, CNAs may help them maintain these qualities. This section will examine real-world instances and situations that can help CNAs provide high-quality care.

Bathing

Maintaining patients' hygiene is an essential part of a CNA's work. Bathing aids might range from overseeing a shower to giving a complete bed bath, depending on the patient's health.

Scenario: Mr. Smith is an old patient who needs help taking a shower because he is not very mobile.

1. Assemble the required materials, including a basin filled with warm water, soap, towels, and washcloths.
2. Make sure the patient is private by drawing curtains or shutting doors.
3. Ask the patient about particular preferences and walk them through the bathing procedure.
4. Help Mr. Smith take off his clothes, making sure he always keeps his dignity intact by using a towel to cover his private parts.
5. One body area at a time, gently wash and rinse with soap and water, and then pat dry with a towel.
6. Help with personal grooming duties like hair combing, shaving, and tooth brushing.
7. Assist Mr. Smith with dressing, keeping his comfort and security in mind.

Feeding

Helping with nutrition and food is another essential part of a CNA's work. They have to ensure patients get all the nutrition they need while honoring their dietary preferences and limitations.

Scenario: Mrs. Johnson needs feeding help during dinner since she is a stroke sufferer who has trouble swallowing.

1. Arrange the dining room to be tidy, free of clutter, and ensure that the patient is positioned comfortably.
2. Wash your hands well, and put on the proper gloves if needed.
3. Check for dietary restrictions or food allergies while describing the meal to Mrs Johnson.
4. Chop meals into bite-sized portions and utilize cutlery that fits her requirements.
5. Give Mrs. Johnson time to herself, and when she needs it, offer encouragement and support.

6. To avoid aspiration or choking, keep an eye on her swallowing and modify the feeding tempo as needed.
7. Keep track of your food and drink consumption and inform the nursing staff if anything seems off.

Mobility

CNAs frequently assist patients with trouble moving around the hospital, ambulating, or transferring from beds to wheelchairs.
Scenario: Mr. Garcia requires assistance getting from his bed to a wheelchair. He is a postoperative patient with restricted mobility.

1. Make sure the wheelchair is fastened into position and that the height of the bed and wheelchair match.
2. Assist Mr. Garcia in sitting on the bed's edge to acclimate briefly.
3. With your feet shoulder-width apart for stability and your knees slightly bent, take a stance facing Mr. Garcia.
4. As you lay your hands on Mr. Garcia's hips, encourage him to place his hands on your shoulders for support.
5. Help Mr. Garcia maintain good body mechanics as he gets up, turns, and lowers himself into the wheelchair.
6. Before releasing the brakes and starting the transfer, ensure Mr. Garcia is snug and secure in the wheelchair.

CNAs assist patients with daily tasks, including eating, dressing, and moving around, which is vital in promoting their general health, independence, and quality of life. CNAs can provide individuals they care for with individualized, sensitive care by comprehending the subtleties of these jobs and using the valuable examples and scenarios discussed in this part.

Toileting and Continence Care

For CNAs, assisting patients with their toileting needs is an essential duty. For patients with incontinence problems, this may entail changing adult briefs, giving bedpans, or helping with bathroom excursions.
Scenario: Mrs. Wilson, the patient, needs her adult briefs changed since she is incontinent.
Gather the required materials, including wipes, adult pants that have been cleaned, gloves, and a plastic bag for disposal.

1. Assure Mrs. Wilson's privacy by shutting doors or drawing curtains as you explain the process.
2. Put Mrs. Wilson on her side, with her back to you, and undo the buttons on the filthy brief.
3. Gently roll the brief in her direction and clean her perineum from front to back with wipes.
4. Once the dirty briefs and wipes have been disposed of, assist Mrs. Wilson in rolling onto her other side so she can clean her behind.
5. Make sure it's tight but not too close by sliding a new adult brief beneath her, adjusting the fit, and fastening the tabs.
6. After using an item, dispose of it appropriately and wash your hands.

Positioning and Turning Patients

Repositioning bedridden individuals regularly helps to maintain circulation and avoid the formation of pressure sores.
Situation: Mr. Brown is a bedridden patient who requires repositioning every two hours.

1. Acquire supplies like extra staff members, a draw sheet, and pillows.
2. Give Mr. Brown an explanation of the process and request his cooperation.
3. Before turning, check for pressure sores or redness on his skin.
4. Adjust the bed to a flat position and loosen any bedding tucked under the mattress.

5. Turn Mr. Brown onto his side and use pillows to keep his body in the correct position.
6. If necessary, use a draw sheet to reduce friction when turning.
7. Every two hours, move Mr. Brown so that the pressure is distributed equally on both sides.

Assisting with Exercise and Range-of-Motion (ROM) Exercises

To preserve their mobility, strength, and flexibility, many patients need help with ROM exercises.
Scenario: Ms. Lee requires assistance with her daily range of motion exercises while she recovers from a hip fracture.

1. Check Ms. Lee's care plan and work with the physical therapist to determine the precise exercises and instructions.
2. Give Ms. Lee an explanation of the exercises, showing her each motion and requesting her cooperation.
3. As Ms. Lee completes the exercises, assist her and, if feasible, encourage her to do it independently.
4. When helping with passive range of motion exercises, carefully and slowly extend each joint to its maximum capacity while paying attention to any pain or discomfort.
5. Track Ms. Lee's development and record any changes or issues so the medical staff knows them.

Social Engagement and Emotional Assistance

CNAs are critical in giving patients who feel alone or vulnerable social connection and emotional support.
Scenario: Mr. Davis, a patient who suffers from loneliness and anxiety, gains from regular company and discussion.

1. Talk with Mr. Davis about things that he finds interesting or have him thinking back on good times.
2. As you actively listen to him, acknowledge his emotions and respond empathetically.
3. Offer to participate in Mr. Davis' favorite pastimes, such as playing cards, watching films, or reading aloud.
4. Urge Mr. Davis to communicate his feelings and, if needed, seek out more assistance from mental health specialists.
5. To promote social interactions, assist in making connections with friends and family via visits or technologies.

Keeping an eye on and reporting condition changes

Because they spend the most time with patients, CNAs are frequently the first to observe changes in their condition. Recognizing and reporting issues as soon as possible can be essential for the patient's welfare.
Scenario: Miss Thompson, a diabetic patient, feels more confused and exhausted than usual.

1. Keep a close eye on Miss Thompson's actions and symptoms and record any changes from her baseline.
2. When reporting your observations to the supervising nurse or healthcare professional
, provide precise and comprehensive information.
3. Work with the medical staff to perform the required interventions, such as monitoring blood sugar levels or modifying medication.
4. Keep an eye on Miss Thompson's health and inform us of any adjustments, gains, or deterioration in her symptoms.
5. Provide Miss Thompson with consolation and emotional support while she works through her health issues.

Assistance with Medication

Licensed nurses are often in charge of giving patients their medications. However, CNAs may also be assigned to remind patients to take their prescriptions or help them with the process.
Scenario: As a patient with hypertension, Mr. Patel needs to take his prescription at certain times of the day.

1. Review Mr. Patel's prescription regimen and ensure you know the right amounts to take at the correct times.
2. Ensure Mr. Patel has water and what he needs, and remind him when to take his prescription.
3. If help is required, offer to open prescription bottles or handle medications.
4. Make sure Mr. Patel has ingested his medication by watching him while he takes it.
5. The record demonstrates that Mr. Patel took his medication as directed and informed the supervising nurse of any problems or worries.

Patient Safety and Fall Prevention

CNAs are essential to keep patients safe and avoid falls, which can result in severe injuries and consequences.
Scenario: Mrs. Robinson is an elderly patient who requires ongoing supervision and aid with mobility due to her high risk of falls.

1. Learn about Mrs. Robinson's fall risk factors and take the necessary precautions, like wearing non-slip shoes, adjusting assistive equipment appropriately, and maintaining a clutter-free environment.
2. When Mrs. Robinson calls for help, remind her to use her call bell and attend to her needs as soon as possible.
3. Help Mrs. Robinson move around while making sure her body is supported, and the mechanics are correct.
4. Keep a watchful eye on her movements, particularly when she moves from sitting to standing or walking.
5. Discuss Mrs. Robinson's fall risk with the medical staff, working together to develop any further interventions or preventative measures.

In conclusion, CNAs need to be proficient in helping patients with everyday tasks to deliver thorough, compassionate care. CNAs can enhance patients' independence, dignity, and well-being by comprehending and putting into practice the real-world examples and scenarios discussed in this part. You may succeed as a CNA and help create a secure and compassionate healthcare environment for everyone by emphasizing clear communication, empathy, and attention to detail.

MONITORING PATIENT CONDITIONS

Although a Certified Nursing Assistant's (CNA) duties are varied, one of the most essential parts of their work is keeping an eye on patients' status and quickly informing medical staff of any changes. CNAs frequently serve as the medical team's eyes and ears, and their vigilance greatly influences patient outcomes. This lengthy part will provide an in-depth discussion of patient condition monitoring and efficient staff-to-staff communication.

A complete grasp of a patient's medical history, including any pre-existing diseases, allergies, and drugs they are taking, is crucial to effectively monitoring their status. Learn about each patient's treatment plan, and if you have any questions or concerns, speak with the supervising nurse.

- **Frequent Evaluation of Vital Signs**. Regularly assessing vital signs, including blood pressure, heart rate, respiration rate, and temperature, is one of the main ways CNAs keep an eye on patients' situations. Ensure you adhere to the frequency specified in the patient's care plan and follow the procedures for taking precise measurements.
- **Looking for Modifications in the Body**. CNAs should be alert in monitoring patients for any physical changes in addition to vital signs. This may involve skin color changes, edema, or improperly healing wounds. Keep an eye out for symptoms of infection, such as discharge, warmth, or redness.
- **Evaluating Emotional and Mental Health**. Monitoring patients' mental and emotional health is equally crucial. Changes in mood, behavior, or cognitive function—such as heightened agitation, confusion, or depression—should be noted by CNAs. Encourage patients to share their thoughts and worries and be there to listen and show empathy.
- **Pain Control and Evaluation**. As a CNA, you'll frequently determine a patient's pain level and ensure they get the right kind of pain medication. Acquire the skill of identifying pain signals in individuals who find it challenging to express their suffering and promptly report any issues to the medical team.
- **Acknowledging and Reporting Adverse Events**. Watch out for side effects, drug interactions, allergies, and other unfavorable reactions to medications or treatments. Report these instances to the medical staff as soon as possible to guarantee that the patient gets the proper attention and care.
- **Record-keeping and Documentation**. For the healthcare team to collaborate and communicate effectively, accurate and current patient observations and care records are essential. Be careful to adhere to the prescribed record-keeping rules while documenting any changes in the patient's status, interventions, and any concerns you may have.
- **Methods of Communication**. It's critical to communicate changes to the medical team clearly, precisely, and concisely. Steer clear of jargon and generalizations in favor of giving precise, in-depth details regarding your observations. When speaking with the medical staff, engage in active listening and be ready to respond to any follow-up inquiries.
- **Developing rapport and trust with patients**. Building rapport and trust with patients is essential for CNAs to monitor their status adequately. This can be accomplished by always giving courteous, kind treatment and having direct, honest conversations. Building strong connections with patients allows CNAs to learn important information about their wants and concerns, which can guide the healthcare team's decision-making.
- **Continuous Learning and Development of Skills**. To keep up with the most recent patient monitoring and reporting standards, CNAs should proactively seek opportunities for continued education and skill development. This could entail signing up for classes, going to workshops, or asking more seasoned coworkers to serve as mentors. Giving your patients the best care possible is possible if you are always learning new things.
- **Changing to Meet the Needs of Each Patient**. Since no two patients are alike, CNAS must be able to modify their observation and reporting methods to suit each patient's particular requirements.

This could be changing how you treat patients with cognitive or communication problems or customizing your techniques to patients with certain cultural or personal preferences.

- **Making Use of Equipment and Technology**. CNAs frequently employ various tools and technology in modern healthcare to help monitor patients' conditions. Please acquaint yourself with the available resources, including vital sign monitors, assistive equipment, and electronic medical record systems, and make sure you know how to utilize them effectively.
- **Assisting Family Members and Careers**. CNAs should actively involve family members and careers in the monitoring and reporting since they are crucial in supporting patients. Openly discuss any changes in the patient's condition with their family and invite them to voice any concerns or observations they may have. CNAs can create a caring and supportive hospital environment by developing a cooperative relationship with patients' loved ones.
- **Maintaining Legal and Ethical Standards**. Maintaining the strictest legal and ethical guidelines is imperative for CNAs to monitor patients' status and inform medical personnel of any changes. This entails protecting patient privacy, getting informed consent where required, and abiding by the rules set forth by your facility and the relevant professional association.
- **Self-Sufficiency and Stress Reduction.** As a CNA can be physically and psychologically demanding, it's imperative to prioritize stress management and self-care. Establish healthy coping strategies and self-care practices to ensure you can provide your patients with the best care possible while still taking care of yourself.

Situation: Mrs. Jackson, a patient with pneumonia, feels her heart racing and her breathlessness suddenly increasing.

1. Examine Mrs. Jackson's medical history and treatment plan, noting any relevant information about her current medications, past medical issues, or recent changes to her regimen.
2. Watch her vitals, including blood pressure, oxygen saturation, and heart rate, and compare them to her predefined baseline.
3. Based on your observations, give a clear and concise explanation of Mrs. Jackson's condition to the supervising nurse or other healthcare expert.
4. Do as instructed if the medical staff tells you to move the patient, give them oxygen, or check their vital signs more often.
5. Monitor
6. Mrs. Jackson's condition and inform the medical personnel of any changes or improvements.

CNAs play a critical role in improving patient safety and well-being by employing a comprehensive approach to monitoring patient conditions and notifying medical staff of any changes. CNAs significantly influence the quality of care provided in healthcare environments because they are committed to excellence, have ongoing education, and develop their skills. Always aim for improvement and growth since the skills and knowledge you acquire will benefit the people you treat.

KNOWLEDGE OF SAFETY PROCEDURES

A Certified Nursing Assistant (CNA) must know about safety protocols and hygienic standards. Following these recommendations helps keep the healthcare environment safe and clean for everyone while ensuring patient well-being. The essential safety precautions and sanitary guidelines that CNAs need to be aware of will be covered in detail in this lengthy section.

- **Hand Hygiene**. Keeping hands clean is one of the most essential parts of a clean healthcare environment. CNAs should use an alcohol-based hand sanitizer if one is not available or wash their hands thoroughly with soap and water for at least 20 seconds. It is recommended to wash your hands before and after handling patients, after coming into contact with potentially contaminated objects, and before putting on and taking off personal protective equipment (PPE).
- **Personal Protective Equipment (PPE)**. PPE is crucial to prevent patients and CNAs from spreading infectious diseases. CNAs must know how to use and discard several personal protective equipment (PPE), including face shields, gloves, masks, and gowns. Ensure you adhere to the policies and procedures set forth by your facility regarding the appropriate times to wear personal protective equipment (PPE) and the safe methods for donning and taking it off.
- **Standard Precautions**. Standard precautions are a collection of infection control procedures that CNAs should follow to stop transmitting contagious diseases. This covers safe injection techniques, handling contaminated materials, respiratory hygiene, cough etiquette, and personal protective equipment (PPE).
- **Transmission-Based Precautions**. When providing care for patients with specific contagious diseases, CNAs should be knowledgeable about transmission-based precautions in addition to standard precautions. These safety measures can be divided into airborne, droplet, and contact precautions. CNAs should be aware of the proper precautions to take for each kind of emergency and adhere to the rules and regulations of their facility.
- **Environmental Cleaning and Disinfection**. Preventing the transmission of infection requires a hygienic and clean healthcare setting. CNAs need to be aware of their responsibilities for keeping the environment clean, including regularly changing sheets, appropriately disposing of trash, and cleaning and sanitizing surfaces.
- **Safe Patient Handling and Mobility**. CNAs help patients move around a lot. Thus, handling patients safely is essential to keep patients and healthcare professionals safe. This entails always adhering to the facility's safety procedures, employing assistance devices when needed, and lifting or transporting patients with appropriate body mechanics.
- **Fall Prevention**. Patients are at a considerable risk of falls, particularly elderly persons and those with limited mobility. CNAs should be familiar with fall prevention techniques, which include making sure the patient's surroundings are safe from potential risks, helping patients move around, and giving them the proper footwear and assistive equipment.
- **Medication Safety**. CNAs should be familiar with the fundamentals of medication safety even if they aren't usually in charge of giving out prescriptions. The "five rights" of medicine administration include the appropriate patient, the right drug, the correct dose, the correct route, and the right time. CNAs can help ensure medication safety by alerting the supervising nurse to any issues or inconsistencies.
- **Emergency Preparedness**. CNAs must be equipped to handle various situations, including medical crises, fires, and natural catastrophes. Learn how to follow the emergency response plan for your facility and where the automated external defibrillators (AEDs) and fire extinguishers are located.
- **Patient Privacy and Confidentiality**. CNAs must abide by the Health Insurance Portability and Accountability Act (HIPAA) and other privacy laws to safeguard patients' private information. This entails keeping patient information confidential, restricting access to medical records, and using caution when exchanging information with other healthcare team members. Regarding patient confidentiality and privacy, always abide by the rules and regulations set forth by your facility.

- **Infection Control**. Keeping the medical environment safe and healthy requires stopping the spread of illnesses. CNAs should be knowledgeable about the telltale signs and symptoms of prevalent ailments as well as the proper protocols for solitary confinement and patient care for patients with communicable diseases. CNAs should also practice good hand hygiene, use personal protective equipment (PPE), and adhere to standard and transmission-based measures.
- **Food Safety and Nutrition**. CNAs must be educated about nutrition and food safety since they help patients prepare meals and feed themselves frequently. This includes being aware of dietary limitations, food allergies, and how crucial a balanced diet is to a patient's health. To avoid a foodborne illness, handle and store food according to the correct procedures.
- **Hazardous Materials and Waste Disposal**. CNAs may encounter dangerous waste in the healthcare industry, including chemicals, sharps, or contaminated linens. Understanding the proper handling and disposal techniques for these items is essential to avoid accidents or environmental contamination. Regarding handling hazardous materials and trash disposal, abide by the rules set forth by your facility and the Occupational Safety and Health Administration (OSHA).
- **Reporting Incidents and Near Misses**. When there is an accident, mistake, or near miss, CNAs should immediately notify their supervisor and finish the necessary paperwork. Open and honest communication can facilitate identifying opportunities for improvement and averting the recurrence of safety issues.
- **Ongoing Education and Training**. As new knowledge and optimal practices become available, safety protocols and hygienic requirements change. To stay current with the most recent standards and guidelines, CNAs should actively pursue continual education and training in safety and hygiene. This could be webinars, workshops, or training sessions tailored to a particular facility.

CNAs who possess a thorough awareness of safety protocols and hygiene standards can contribute to the establishment of a safe and healthy healthcare environment for patients and staff. Your diligent adherence to these rules and ongoing acquisition of new knowledge in these areas as a Certified Nursing Assistant will significantly impact patient care and general facility safety. It's important to stay current with the most recent advice and recognize and take proactive measures to resolve any potential safety risks.

EFFECTIVE COMMUNICATION WITH PATIENTS, FAMILIES, AND HEALTHCARE STAFF

Good communication is crucial for a Certified Nursing Assistant (CNA) to provide patients with high-quality care and to create a healthy work environment with coworkers. This comprehensive section will examine many facets of successful communication, emphasizing how CNAs can interact with patients, families, and medical personnel.

- **Active Listening**. A key element of good communication is active listening. Giving the speaker your undivided attention, refraining from interruptions, and, if needed, seeking clarification are all examples of active listening. In addition to assisting you in understanding the speaker's point of view, active listening shows that you genuinely care about their issues.
- **Empathy and Compassion**. Building a relationship and earning the trust of patients and their families requires empathy and compassion. Show kindness by confirming the patient's feelings, recognizing their emotions, and genuinely caring about their welfare. Demonstrating empathy and compassion can reduce anxiety and promote a good rapport between the patient and the career.
- **Verbal Communication**. CNAs must be able to communicate verbally while discussing patient care, updating family members, or working with other CNAs. Try to speak intelligibly and succinctly, using suitable language, and have a polite and formal tone. To guarantee understanding, consider the patient's or family's degree of health literacy and modify your wording accordingly.
- **Nonverbal Communication**
- Nonverbal cues, including body language, gestures, and facial expressions, can significantly influence our messages. When interacting with patients, families, and coworkers, remember your nonverbal clues and keep an open, welcoming body language. When appropriate, smile, make eye contact, and refrain from crossing your arms or projecting a lack of interest.
- **Cultural Sensitivity**. CNAs must be attentive to cultural differences when interacting with patients and families in today's diverse healthcare environment. This entails honoring cultural customs, being cognizant of any communication gaps, and, if practical, making accommodations for personal or religious preferences. It can guarantee successful communication and foster an inclusive healthcare environment by exhibiting cultural awareness.
- **Patient Education**. CNAs are critical in teaching patients and their families about many facets of their treatment, including managing their sickness, taking their medications, and caring for themselves. When educating patients, speak clearly; avoid medical jargon. When appropriate, provide written materials or visual aids to enhance knowledge and encourage inquiries.
- **Conflict Resolution**. CNAs should be ready to handle conflicts between patients, relatives, and medical personnel professionally and effectively. When faced with disagreements, keep your composure and objectivity, pay attention to everyone, and cooperate to find a solution. Apply a supervisor or other suitable team member to assist in mediating the conflict, if necessary.
- **Therapeutic Communication Techniques**. Therapeutic communication is a specific method of interacting with patients that enhances emotional health and creates a caring environment. CNAs should know various therapeutic communication strategies, including asking open-ended questions, considering the patient's emotions, and offering consolation and support.
- **Documentation and Reporting**. Good communication in the healthcare setting depends on accurate reporting and recording. CNAs are responsible for making sure that all observations, interventions, and activities related to patient care are wholly and accurately recorded in the patient's medical file. Furthermore, CNAs are responsible for promptly informing the relevant healthcare team members of any changes in the patient's status or concerns.
- **Interprofessional Collaboration.** CNAs collaborate closely with various medical specialists, such as social workers, therapists, doctors, and nurses. The coordination of patient care and the

assurance that all team members know the patient's requirements and progress depend heavily on effective interprofessional communication. To promote effective interprofessional collaboration, CNAs should proactively exchange information, actively engage in team meetings, and solicit advice from peers as needed.

- **Telephone and Electronic Communication**. Telephone and electronic communication are essential for sustaining efficient communication between healthcare team members, patients, and families in the modern healthcare setting. CNAs should know how to use email, phone systems, and other electronic communication tools safely and securely while abiding by confidentiality and privacy laws. Keep your communication clear, professional, and kind when using technological means.

- **Family Meetings and Care Conferences.** CNAs may be required to participate in family meetings or care conferences to discuss a patient's care plan and progress. CNAs should be ready to discuss observations, provide updates on the patient's status, and provide feedback on possible care plans during these meetings. Have open lines of communication with every team member and treat the patient and their family with respect and support.

- **Patient Advocacy**. One of your responsibilities as a CNA is to advocate for your patients, ensuring the medical staff listens to them and respects their choices. When required, speak up for your patients' interests and cooperate with other team members to guarantee patient-centered care.

- **Communication Challenges and Strategies**. CNAs may have trouble communicating with patients with cognitive, speech, or hearing problems. Learn about the several communication techniques and assistive technology that can help you communicate more effectively, such as picture boards, communication apps, and hearing aids.

- **Self-Reflection and Growth**. Strive for constant improvement in your communication abilities by asking patients, relatives, and coworkers for input. Determine your areas of weakness and work on them through courses, workshops, or mentoring programs to strengthen your communication skills.

In summary, good communication is an essential CNA ability needed to provide high-quality patient care and a positive healthcare environment.

CNAs can successfully work with family members and colleagues, improve communication skills, and better meet the requirements of their patients by putting the methods and practices described in this extensive guide into practice. You should always aim to get better at communicating and be willing to learn new things and develop this crucial part of your job as a CNA.

ADVANCED PATIENT CARE TECHNIQUES FOR CNAS

Welcome to the heart of your journey toward becoming an exceptional Certified Nursing Assistant. This chapter will take your learning to new heights as we delve into 'Advanced Patient Care Techniques for CNAs.' As a CNA, your role extends beyond primary care. Your knowledge and skills are essential in enhancing the health and well-being of the patients you serve. This chapter dives deeper into specialized care practices, focusing on the advanced techniques that set seasoned CNAs apart from beginners. We'll cover some critical subjects: wound management, specialist treatment for chronic illnesses, palliative and hospice care, geriatric care and dementia support, and rehabilitation and restorative care.

Each of these topics is crucial to providing comprehensive patient care, and understanding them will equip you with the knowledge and abilities required to provide the most excellent care for your patients.

We'll also discuss leadership, teamwork, and advanced communication skills, emphasizing the importance of these traits in the quick-paced healthcare sector. Skills in cooperation and effective communication are crucial since they significantly impact the quality of treatment you can provide patients.

By the end of this chapter, you'll be more knowledgeable about the most recent advancements in patient care and equipped with the abilities you need to handle difficult circumstances as your career progresses. To significantly enhance the lives of our patients, let's get ready and learn more about advanced care.

Management of wound care

For CNAs caring for patients with acute or chronic wounds, managing wound care is a critical component of patient care. The greatest patient outcomes depend on understanding different forms of damage, wound healing concepts, and sophisticated wound care approaches.

The following are some of the wounds that CNAs could experience:

- **Abrasions:** These are superficial wounds that only affect the skin's surface layers and are brought on by friction or scraping.
- **Lacerations:** These are deeper skin tears or cuts that may include underlying tissues and structures. They are frequently brought on by accidents or the usage of sharp tools.
- **Puncture** wounds are wounds caused by a sharp item, like a needle or a nail, piercing the skin.
- **Incisions:** These are neat, straight cuts that typically appear after surgery.
- **Contusions:** Also referred to as bruises, these are brought on by a blow to the body that affects the blood vessels under the skin.
- **Burns:** These injuries can range in severity from superficial to full-thickness and are brought on by heat, chemicals, or radiation.

The first stage of stopping bleeding is called hemostasis, during which blood vessels constrict and clotting factors are activated.

- **Inflammation:** During this phase, immune cells such as white blood cells and others go to the site of the wound to eliminate bacteria and remove debris.
- **Proliferation:** In the wound bed, new blood vessels and granulation tissue appear. Cells called fibroblasts also make collagen to fortify the tissue.
- **Restructuring:** The last step, which can take months or even years to complete, entails restructuring collagen fibers and producing scar tissue.

Advanced wound care techniques
- **Dressing changes:** CNAs should follow the healthcare provider's instructions for dressing changes, including the type of dressing, frequency, and technique. CNAs should use aseptic techniques to

prevent infection when changing dressings and always wear gloves. They should also assess the wound for signs of infection or complications, such as increased redness, swelling, or discharge.

- **Wound assessment:** Regular wound assessment is essential for monitoring healing progress and detecting potential issues. CNAs should note the size, depth, color, and appearance of the wound, as well as the condition of the surrounding skin. They should also document any pain or discomfort the patient experiences.
- **Prevention of infection:** Maintaining a clean and sterile environment is crucial for preventing wound infections. CNAs should practice hand hygiene, wear gloves, and use sterile instruments and dressings when handling wounds. They should also educate patients and their families on the importance of keeping the damage clean and dry and promptly report any signs of infection.
- **Debridement:** In some cases, removing dead or infected tissue (debridement) may be necessary to promote wound healing. A qualified healthcare professional should only perform this procedure.
- **Negative pressure wound therapy (NPWT):** For complex or hard-to-heal wounds, NPWT may be used. This involves applying a vacuum device to the injury, which helps remove excess fluid, reduce bacteria, and promote granulation tissue formation. CNAs may monitor the device and assist with dressing changes during NPWT.

In conclusion, CNAs play a vital role in wound care management. By understanding the types of wounds, principles of wound healing, and advanced wound care techniques, they can provide the best possible care for their patients and help prevent complications associated with wound healing.

Specialized care for chronic conditions

Caring for patients with chronic conditions presents unique challenges and requires specialized knowledge and skills from CNAs. By understanding the specific care requirements associated with common chronic illnesses, such as diabetes, COPD, and Parkinson's disease, CNAs can provide tailored support to improve the quality of life for these patients.

Diabetes

Diabetes is a chronic condition characterized by elevated blood sugar levels due to the body's inability to produce or effectively use insulin. CNAs should be aware of the following aspects when caring for diabetic patients:

- **Blood glucose monitoring:** CNAs may assist with blood glucose testing, ensuring patients perform tests regularly and accurately. They should also be familiar with the target glucose ranges and recognize signs of high or low blood sugar, such as dizziness, confusion, or sweating.
- **Medication management:** CNAs may help diabetic patients with medication administration, including oral medications and insulin injections. It is essential to ensure that patients take their medications as prescribed and are aware of potential side effects or interactions.
- **Nutrition and meal planning:** CNAs can support diabetic patients by guiding meal planning, portion control, and healthy food choices, as well as monitoring their carbohydrate intake. They should also know the importance of regular meal schedules to maintain stable blood sugar levels.
- **Foot care:** Diabetic patients risk developing foot complications due to poor circulation and nerve damage. CNAs should regularly inspect the patient's feet for cuts, blisters, or signs of infection and encourage proper foot hygiene and footwear.

COPD (Chronic Obstructive Pulmonary Disease)

COPD is a group of lung diseases, including chronic bronchitis and emphysema, which cause breathing difficulties. CNAs should consider the following when caring for patients with COPD:

- **Breathing exercises and techniques:** CNAs can teach patients with COPD various breathing techniques, such as pursed-lip breathing and diaphragmatic breathing, to help them manage shortness of breath.
- **Oxygen therapy:** CNAs may administer and monitor oxygen therapy for COPD patients. This includes ensuring the equipment functions correctly, adjusting the flow rate as needed, and watching the patient for signs of oxygen toxicity or other complications.
- **Medication management:** CNAs should be familiar with the medications commonly prescribed for COPD, such as bronchodilators and corticosteroids, and assist patients with proper administration.
- **Energy conservation:** CNAs can help COPD patients conserve energy by encouraging them to pace themselves during daily activities, take regular breaks, and prioritize essential tasks.

Parkinson's disease

Parkinson's disease is a progressive neurological disorder that affects movement and coordination. CNAs should be mindful of the following when caring for patients with Parkinson's disease:

- **Mobility assistance:** CNAs can provide support with walking, transfers, and balance exercises to help Parkinson's patients maintain mobility and prevent falls.
- **Communication support:** CNAs should be patient and attentive when communicating with Parkinson's patients, as they may have difficulty speaking or expressing themselves. Simple, explicit language and ample time for the patient to respond can facilitate better communication.
- **Management of medications:** CNAs need to be knowledgeable about the drugs used to treat Parkinson's disease, such as levodopa and dopamine agonists, and ensure patients take them as directed. They should watch for changes in the patient's health and be mindful of any adverse effects.
- **Support for swallowing and nutrition:** CNAs may help Parkinson's patients during mealtime by urging them to take tiny bites, eat slowly, and keep an upright posture to avoid choking. Additionally, they should monitor the patient's nutritional condition and address issues like weight loss or trouble chewing.

Support for emotional and mental health

CNAs should be aware that a chronic illness can impact a patient's emotional and mental health. The patient's attitude and resilience may be significantly affected by listening to them, encouraging them, and creating a supportive environment.

- **Treatment coordination:** To guarantee that patients with chronic diseases receive the most appropriate
- and thorough treatment possible, CNAs may work with other healthcare professionals, including doctors, nurses, therapists, and nutritionists. This includes exchanging observations and worries, participating in care-planning sessions, and carrying out care-plan interventions.
- **Patient education:** CNAs should thoroughly understand the chronic illnesses they deal with and be ready to inform patients and their families about the condition's symptoms, available treatments, and self-care techniques. Patients can be empowered to actively manage their needs and make knowledgeable decisions about their care by being given accurate and pertinent information.
- **Adjusting to changing demands:** Patients' needs could alter over time as chronic illnesses worsen. CNAs should be ready to modify their care strategy as necessary and to regularly monitor the patient's state to spot any emerging problems or issues.

In conclusion, CNAs are critical in providing patients with chronic diseases with specialized care. CNAs can help these patients live more comfortable, fulfilled lives while managing their condition by having a comprehensive grasp of the distinctive elements of each illness and improving their abilities in areas including wound care, mobility aid, medication administration, and patient education.

Palliative and hospice care

Patients and their families receiving palliative and hospice care are supported. Understanding the guiding concepts behind these care strategies, your responsibility for offering consolation and support, and the finest end-of-life care procedures can help you as a CNA provide better care for patients and their loved ones during this trying time.

- **Palliative care guiding principles:** Patients with severe or terminal diseases can benefit from palliative care by reducing their suffering and improving their quality of life. This compassionate method aims to help patients and their families while controlling symptoms and attending to emotional and spiritual needs. Palliative care can be given alongside curative therapies at any stage of severe disease, not just in cases where a patient is nearing death.
- **Hospice care:** Hospice care is a subset of palliative care that focuses on giving patients with terminal diagnoses compassionate end-of-life care. Hospice care ensures that patients have a peaceful and dignified dying, supported by medical experts and present with their loved ones. Typically, hospice care is given at the patient's home or a designated hospice facility.
- **CNAs' role in hospice and palliative care:** The calming and hospice care teams depend heavily on CNAs. They give patients direct care, such as aid with everyday tasks like mobility and personal hygiene, all while keeping an eye out for changes in the patient's conditions. Additionally, CNAs provide patients and their families with emotional support and company, which helps to foster a soothing and encouraging environment.
- **Managing symptoms:** Controlling physical symptoms, including pain, nausea, exhaustion, and shortness of breath, is an essential part of palliative and hospice care. CNAs can aid by giving medicine as directed, helping with non-pharmacological therapies like positioning and massage, and alerting the care team immediately if any symptoms go out of control.
- **Support for patients' emotional and spiritual needs:** CNAs may help patients and their families with their emotional and spiritual needs by listening to them, encouraging them, and enabling access to spiritual care providers like chaplains, counselors, or support groups.
- **Family support:** CNAs can help families deal with the difficulties of caring for a loved one with a life-limiting disease by providing them with practical aid and emotional support. This can be supplying respite care, helping with chores around the house, or lending a shoulder when things get tough.
- **Best practices for end-of-life care:** As patients get closer to passing away, CNAs need to know the best ways to give them empathetic, dignified care. This entails identifying the warning indications of imminent death, preserving the patient's physical comfort, offering the patient and their family emotional support, and honoring their cultural and spiritual customs.

In conclusion, CNAs are crucial in delivering hospice and palliative care to patients and their families suffering from life-limiting illnesses. CNAs may significantly impact the lives of persons they care for during this trying time by comprehending the guiding concepts of these care approaches, gaining the ability to manage symptoms and offer emotional support, and following best practices for end-of-life care.

Geriatric care and dementia support

Given that older persons frequently need specialized care because of their particular health difficulties, geriatric care, and dementia assistance are crucial specialties for CNAs. CNAs may enhance the quality of life for older adults and their families by learning advanced strategies for controlling behavioral symptoms, offering emotional support, and attending to the particular requirements of dementia patients.

- **Understanding the aging process:** CNAs need to know how aging often affects a person's physical and mental capabilities to offer good geriatric care. With this knowledge, CNAs can distinguish between changes in a patient's condition brought on by normal aging and those that could indicate a severe health problem.
- **Managing behavioral symptoms:** Agitation, anger, and roaming are behavioral symptoms that older persons, especially those with dementia, may display. CNAs can assist in addressing these symptoms by establishing a controlled and predictable environment, employing tactful redirection and validation tactics, and swiftly alerting the care team to any troubling behaviors.
- **Offering emotional support:** As their health, living condition, or social support network change, older persons may feel loneliness, sadness, and anxiety. By engaging patients in deep discussion, providing company, and promoting social interaction, CNAs may help patients emotionally.
- **Addressing the particular difficulties experienced by dementia patients**: People with dementia may have cognitive decline, memory loss, and communication issues, which make daily chores difficult. Clear and direct communication, signals and reminders for everyday duties, and modifying one's approach to suit the patient's changing requirements are all ways that CNAs may help these patients.
- **Supporting independence and autonomy:** Older persons may need help with everyday tasks, but it's crucial to support freedom and independence wherever feasible. CNAs may offer enough assistance to keep patients safe while letting them do things independently, promoting a sense of success and self-worth.
- **Ensuring safety:** Due to age-related changes in movement, balance, and eyesight, older persons may be more susceptible to falls, accidents, and injuries. By eliminating hazards, making use of assistive equipment when necessary, and attentively watching patients for indications of increased fall risk, CNAs contribute to maintaining a safe workplace.
- **Recognizing and combating elder abuse:** Unfortunately, older persons might be particularly susceptible to neglect and financial, emotional, and physical abuse. Elder abuse must be identified by CNAs, who must also report any suspicions to the proper authorities.
- **Collaborating with the healthcare team:** Providing comprehensive geriatric care and dementia support requires collaboration among various healthcare professionals, such as physicians, nurses, social workers, and therapists. CNAs should communicate openly with the care team, share relevant observations, and seek guidance when needed.

In summary, CNAs are vital in providing geriatric care and dementia support to older adults. By developing advanced skills in managing behavioral symptoms, providing emotional support, and addressing the unique challenges faced by dementia patients, CNAs can help improve the quality of life for older adults and their families. Continual learning and collaboration with the healthcare team will further enhance the ability of CNAs to meet the complex needs of this population.

Rehabilitation and restorative care

Rehabilitation and restorative care are critical in helping patients regain their independence and return to their daily activities after an illness, injury, or surgery. CNAs are essential rehabilitation team members, assisting patients with physical therapy exercises, mobility training and promoting independence throughout recovery. The following are critical aspects of rehabilitation and restorative care in which CNAs can make a significant impact:

- **Understanding the rehabilitation goals:** CNAs should familiarize themselves with each patient's rehabilitation goals and the care plan developed by the healthcare team. This understanding will help CNAs provide appropriate support and encouragement to patients as they work towards regaining their abilities.

- **Assisting with physical therapy exercises:** CNAs may work closely with physical therapists to help patients perform prescribed activities to improve strength, flexibility, balance, and coordination. CNAs can ensure patient safety during exercises, assist as needed, and offer encouragement and motivation to help patients achieve their rehabilitation goals.
- **Mobility training:** CNAs play a crucial role in helping patients regain mobility, whether learning to walk again or using assistive devices such as walkers or wheelchairs. CNAs can support patients by providing physical assistance, monitoring for signs of fatigue or discomfort, and ensuring a safe environment for mobility training.
- **Promoting independence:** CNAs should encourage patients to actively participate in their recovery and perform tasks independently whenever possible throughout the rehabilitation process. This approach can boost patients' confidence, self-esteem, and motivation to continue working toward their rehabilitation goals.
- **Providing emotional support:** Rehabilitation can be challenging and dynamic for patients who may experience frustration, sadness, or fear. CNAs can provide emotional support by listening to patients' concerns, offering empathy and understanding, and reinforcing their progress.
- **Monitoring progress and reporting changes:** CNAs should closely observe patients during rehabilitation and report any changes in their abilities, pain levels, or emotional well-being to the healthcare team. This ongoing communication helps adjust the care plan to support the patient's recovery best.
- **Supporting patients with adaptive equipment:** CNAs may assist patients in using adaptive equipment, such as grab bars, raised toilet seats, or shower chairs, to promote independence and safety during daily activities. CNAs should be familiar with these devices' proper use and maintenance to provide adequate support.
- **Education and self-care:** CNAs can play a vital role in educating patients and their families about self-care techniques, such as proper body mechanics, energy conservation strategies, and home safety modifications. This knowledge can empower patients to take control of their recovery and reduce the risk of injury or setbacks.

In conclusion, CNAs are crucial in rehabilitation and restorative care, providing valuable support to patients as they regain their independence and abilities. CNAs can significantly impact patients' recovery and overall well-being by assisting with physical therapy exercises, mobility training, and promoting independence. Ongoing education and collaboration with the healthcare team will further enhance the CNAs' ability to provide practical, patient-centered care during rehabilitation.

Advanced communication skills

Advanced communication skills are essential for CNAs to navigate complex and challenging situations effectively. These skills can help CNAs build strong relationships with patients, families, and healthcare team members, ultimately improving patient outcomes and enhancing the healthcare experience. This section will explore practical strategies for addressing concerns, providing education, and managing conflicts in various settings.

- **Active listening:** Active listening is a critical component of effective communication. It involves giving the speaker your full attention, maintaining eye contact, nodding, and using verbal and non-verbal cues to show you are engaged. Active listening helps establish trust, fosters empathy, and enables you to understand the speaker's feelings, concerns, and needs.
- **Empathy and compassion:** 2. Empathy and compassion: Being friendly and compassionate toward patients, families, and coworkers is essential. Putting yourself in their situation can help you better understand their feelings and experiences, improving your ability to respond and offer the proper assistance.
- **Clear and succinct communication:** It's crucial to be precise and concise while giving directions or delivering information. Ensure the listener gets the message by using clear language and avoiding jargon. Asking them to repeat the details or rules can help you ensure they understand.
- **Addressing worries:** When patients or family members voice concerns, they must pay close attention, acknowledge their emotions, and reassure them. Give them information and resources

that can help them with their issues, and, as necessary, include other healthcare team members to ensure proper follow-up and support.

- **Teaching patients and families:** CNAs have a big part to play in teaching patients and families about many elements of care, such as treatment plans, self-care strategies, and lifestyle changes. Present information succinctly and coherently, utilizing visual aids or demonstrations as necessary to successfully educate people. To ensure the information is conveyed clearly, ask questions and check for understanding.
- **Conflict resolution:** Various factors, including poor communication, divergent viewpoints, and high-stress circumstances, can lead to conflicts in healthcare settings. Maintaining composure while listening to all parties involved and trying to understand their views can help you manage disagreements effectively. Directly address the problem and identify a workable solution for all parties. Apply a manager or other team members to mediate and settle the dispute.
- **Cultural sensitivity:** Because healthcare environments vary widely, CNAs must interact successfully with patients, families, and coworkers from various cultural backgrounds. Learn about other cultures, traditions, and communication styles, then use this information in your relationships to become more culturally competent. Be courteous, open-minded, and willing to change your approach to promote clear communication and comprehension.
- **Nonverbal communication**: Nonverbal clues like body language, gestures, and facial expressions may send solid messages and affect how well you communicate. Be conscious of your nonverbal clues and make sure they support the message you want to convey. Please also be mindful of others' nonverbal signs since these might reveal important information about their emotions and worries.
- **Collaboration and teamwork:** Good collaboration and partnership are built on effective communication in healthcare settings. Openly exchange information, take in other people's opinions and work on solutions as a group. Healthcare personnel may deliver excellent patient care and support one another in trying circumstances by working as a cohesive team.
- **Maintaining professional boundaries:** CNAs must establish and maintain appropriate professional boundaries with patients, families, and colleagues. These boundaries help ensure that relationships remain focused on the patient's best interests and maintain a professional and therapeutic environment. Be aware of potential boundary violations, such as developing personal relationships with patients or engaging in inappropriate discussions. Always keep a professional demeanor and adhere to established guidelines and ethical standards.
- **Developing assertiveness:** Assertiveness is an essential communication skill that allows CNAs to express their needs, opinions, and concerns respectfully and honestly. Growing emphasis can help CNAs advocate for themselves and their patients while maintaining positive relationships with healthcare team members. Practice assertiveness by using "I" statements, maintaining eye contact, and using a confident tone when expressing your thoughts and feelings.
- **Utilizing appropriate communication channels:** In a healthcare setting, there are various communication channels available for sharing information, such as face-to-face conversations, phone calls, emails, and electronic medical records. Understand the appropriate use of each communication channel and effectively convey essential information to the relevant parties. Be mindful of privacy and confidentiality concerns, and ensure that sensitive data is shared only with those who need to know.
- **Time management and organization:** Effective communication also involves managing time and organizing information efficiently. Develop time management skills by prioritizing tasks, setting goals, and using tools such as to-do lists and schedules. Organize information systematically, using tools such as electronic health records or care plans, to facilitate effective communication with healthcare team members.
- **Seeking feedback and continuous improvement:** To enhance your communication skills, seek input from patients, families, and colleagues, and use it to identify areas for improvement. Engage in self-reflection and strive for continuous growth by attending workshops, participating in training sessions, and staying informed about best communication practices.

In summary, CNAs play a vital role in healthcare settings, and practical communication skills are essential for providing high-quality care and support to patients and families. By focusing on active listening, empathy, cultural competence, and conflict resolution, CNAs can easily navigate complex and challenging situations. Developing assertiveness, maintaining professional boundaries, and utilizing appropriate communication channels will further enhance CNAs' ability to foster positive relationships with patients, families, and healthcare team members. Finally, CNAs can ensure they continue to grow and excel in their roles by seeking feedback and engaging in continuous improvement.

Leadership and teamwork

Explore the importance of leadership and teamwork in the CNA role, including strategies for effective collaboration, delegation, and decision-making within a healthcare team.

- **Understanding the role of a CNA leader:** While CNAs may not hold formal leadership positions, they can still exhibit leadership qualities in their daily work. A CNA leader demonstrates initiative, takes responsibility, and is a role model for their peers. They consistently display professionalism, excellent communication skills, and a commitment to high-quality patient care.
- **Creating a positive team environment:** A positive team environment encourages cooperation, mutual trust, and respect among healthcare team members. By being encouraging, courteous, and understanding toward their coworkers as well as by recognizing and appreciating the accomplishments of others, CNAs may help to create a healthy culture. The dynamics of a team may also be improved by promoting free communication and giving helpful criticism.
- **Active engagement in interprofessional team meetings:** CNAs should actively engage in interprofessional team meetings, contributing their knowledge, observations, and experience to guide planning and decision-making for patient care. By participating in these conversations, CNAs make ensuring that patient care plans are thorough, unique, and built on a full grasp of the patient's requirements and preferences.
- **Effective task delegation and management:** CNAs frequently collaborate with other nursing staff members, such as licensed practical nurses (LPNs) and registered nurses (RNs), and they could be given tasks to accomplish as part of the patient care plan. To ensure that tasks are allocated and carried out quickly and effectively, it is essential to understand the fundamentals of successful delegation and task management. This entails comprehending the range of one's work, setting priorities, and keeping lines of communication open with colleagues.
- **Conflict resolution and problem-solving**: Disagreements and disputes can occur in any team environment. To resolve these conflicts amicably and uphold a productive workplace, CNAs must have conflict resolution and problem-solving abilities. Active listening, understanding others' viewpoints, and seeking compromise are all skills that may be used to settle disputes and foster unity among the members of the healthcare team.
- **Adaptability and flexibility:** Because the healthcare industry is always evolving, CNAs need to be flexible in how they approach providing patient care and collaborating with others. This entails being adaptable to shifting schedules or care plans, welcoming chances for learning and development, and remaining open to new ideas.
- **Cultivating leadership skills:** While not every CNA may aspire to a formal leadership role, acquiring leadership skills can enhance personal and professional development. CNAs can pursue continuing education opportunities, such as workshops and seminars, to develop communication, problem-solving, and decision-making skills. Additionally, seeking mentorship from experienced CNAs or nursing professionals can provide valuable insights and guidance.
- **Advocacy for patients and colleagues:** CNAs play a critical role in advocating for their patient's needs and well-being and supporting their colleagues. This may involve speaking up when a patient's care plan needs adjustment or advocating for additional resources to support patient care. By actively advocating for patients and colleagues, CNAs can help ensure the delivery of high-quality, patient-centered care.

In conclusion, leadership and teamwork are vital components of a successful CNA career. By developing communication, conflict resolution, and collaboration skills, CNAs can contribute to a positive, supportive healthcare team environment that promotes high-quality patient care. Embracing opportunities for growth and learning can further enhance CNAs' leadership capabilities and professional development.

CNA EXAM AND REQUIREMENTS

To embark on your journey toward becoming a Certified Nursing Assistant (CNA), it's vital to grasp the intricacies and structure of the CNA exam. This chapter aims to provide a comprehensive overview of the CNA test, encompassing its components, prerequisites, and eligibility criteria. Additionally, we will delve into the registration process and offer strategies for success.

The CNA exam typically comprises two main segments: a written (or oral) test and a skills assessment. The written test consists of multiple-choice questions encompassing various topics related to the duties and responsibilities of nursing assistants. These subjects include fundamental nursing principles, patient care, communication skills, and safety protocols. In some states, an oral version of the exam may be available if an applicant faces challenges in reading English or has recognized impairments that hinder them from completing a written test.

On the other hand, the skills evaluation component assesses your practical proficiency in a spectrum of nursing assistant tasks. These tasks may encompass hand hygiene, patient transfers, and the accurate measurement of vital signs. During the skills exam, candidates must demonstrate a specific number of competencies chosen from a predetermined list. To enhance your confidence and competence, it is imperative to familiarize yourself with the skills that could be evaluated during the exam and consistently practice them. Understanding these fundamental aspects of the CNA exam is a crucial first step toward achieving success in becoming a Certified Nursing Assistant.

Conditions for the CNA Exam

Before pursuing a Certified Nursing Assistant (CNA) career, you must understand the conditions you must meet to qualify for the CNA exam. To become eligible, you need a high school diploma or its equivalent, a clean criminal background check, and the successful completion of a state-approved CNA training program. These training programs typically consist of both classroom instruction and hands-on clinical training, ensuring you acquire the necessary knowledge and skills to provide competent patient care.

In addition to educational requirements, candidates must often provide proof of immunizations and undergo a health screening to ensure they are physically fit for the job's demands. The specifics of these conditions may vary from state to state, so it's crucial to consult your state's nursing board or regulatory agency for precise guidelines.

Enrolling for the CNA Exam

Once you've met the necessary conditions, the next step is enrolling for the CNA exam. This process typically involves submitting an application, paying an exam fee, and scheduling your test date. It's essential to be aware of the application deadlines and requirements specific to your state, as there can be variations in the application process.

Many states utilize the National Nurse Aide Assessment Program (NNAAP) exam, which consists of a written or oral test and a practical skills evaluation. To ensure you secure your preferred exam date, it's advisable to apply well in advance, as testing centers may have limited availability.

CNA Exam Preparation

Preparing for the CNA exam is a critical step toward success. Begin by thoroughly reviewing the materials covered during your training program, including class notes, textbooks, and training manuals. Consider utilizing CNA exam preparation books or online resources that offer practice tests and sample questions.

Familiarizing yourself with the exam format, which includes written/oral and practical skills evaluations, is crucial. For the skills evaluation portion, practice essential CNA skills such as taking vital signs, assisting with activities of daily living, and following infection control procedures. Confidence and competence during the practical assessment are essential for a positive outcome.

Exam Day Advice and Techniques

On the day of the CNA exam, being well-prepared and composed is essential. Ensure that you arrive well-rested and ready to tackle the challenges ahead. Dress in a professional and appropriate CNA uniform, and remember to bring two forms of identification as required. Read each question carefully during the written or oral test, take your time, and avoid rushing through the exam. Proper time management is crucial to ensure ample time to complete all sections.

For the skills evaluation, adhere to the correct procedures step by step. Maintain effective communication with the "patient," who is typically an evaluator, and exhibit a calm and professional demeanor throughout the examination. Remember to prioritize patient safety and practice stringent infection control measures.

Getting Your Exam Results and Certification

After completing the CNA exam, you can expect to receive your results within a few weeks. If you pass both the written/oral and skills evaluations, you can apply for CNA certification. Your state's nursing board or regulatory agency will issue your certification, which officially permits you to work as a CNA in your state.

Keeping up with and Renewing Your CNA Credentials

To maintain your CNA credentials and continue working in this valuable healthcare profession, staying informed about your state's renewal requirements is essential. These requirements typically involve completing a specified number of continuing education hours and providing evidence of ongoing employment as a CNA. Renewing your certification on time ensures that you remain current in your knowledge and skills, enabling you to provide the best possible care to your patients.

Analyzing the CNA Exam Questions in Detail

Understanding the types of questions encountered in the written (or oral) test and the skills evaluation is crucial for success on the Certified Nursing Assistant (CNA) exam. This chapter aims to comprehensively examine the question formats and subject areas covered on the CNA test to prepare candidates better.

Questions for the Written (or Oral) Examination

The written (or oral) examination segment of the CNA exam typically comprises 60 to 100 multiple-choice questions, depending on the state and testing organization. These questions assess candidates' knowledge of various topics related to the responsibilities and tasks of a nursing assistant. These topics can be broadly categorized as follows:

1. Basic Nursing Principles: This category encompasses questions related to fundamental nursing principles, including infection control, proper body mechanics, and appropriate patient positioning. Candidates may be asked about personal protective equipment (PPE), methods for preventing disease transmission, and safe techniques for moving and transferring patients.

2. Patient Care: This section includes questions about the routine care of patients, covering activities such as grooming, feeding, toileting, and bathing. Candidates can expect inquiries about the correct procedures for assisting patients with personal hygiene, maintaining privacy and dignity while delivering care, and ensuring patients' nutritional needs are met.

3. Communication: Questions in this category assess candidates' ability to communicate effectively with patients, their families, and fellow healthcare professionals. Topics may include active listening skills, verbal and nonverbal communication techniques, and strategies for dealing with challenging communication situations, such as working with patients with cognitive impairments or language barriers.

4. Safety Procedures: This area focuses on questions related to maintaining a safe environment for patients and healthcare personnel. Topics may include fall prevention strategies, emergency preparedness protocols, and fire safety procedures.

5. Legal and Ethical Issues: Questions in this category revolve around the legal and ethical responsibilities of CNAs, including patient rights, confidentiality, and mandatory reporting. Candidates might be quizzed on specific laws and regulations about nursing assistants and the ethical considerations involved in making decisions in healthcare settings.

6. Mental Health and Psychosocial Needs: This category addresses questions related to addressing patients' emotional and psychosocial needs. Topics may include strategies for managing behavioral challenges, providing emotional support, and coping mechanisms for individuals dealing with stress, anxiety, or depression.

Skills Evaluation Questions

The skills evaluation portion of the CNA exam is a practical assessment of a candidate's ability to perform various nursing assistant tasks. Candidates are typically required to demonstrate a set number of skills (often 3 to 5) chosen by the evaluator from a predetermined list.

Some specific skills that may be evaluated during the skills assessment include:

1. Hand Hygiene: Candidates are assessed on their ability to perform proper handwashing techniques and understand the importance of hand hygiene in preventing the spread of infections.

2. Vital Signs Measurement: Candidates must accurately measure a patient's vital signs, including blood pressure, pulse rate, respiratory rate, and temperature, and record these measurements correctly.

3. Patient Transfers: This skill evaluates candidates' proficiency in assisting patients with safe transfers between surfaces (e.g., bed to wheelchair) using appropriate body mechanics and transfer techniques.

4. Bed Making: Candidates are assessed on their ability to make a bed correctly, whether occupied or unoccupied, to ensure patient comfort and maintain a clean and safe environment.

5. Personal Protective Equipment (PPE): This skill assesses candidates' knowledge of correctly donning and doffing personal protective equipment (PPE) to protect themselves and their patients from infections. PPE includes items like gloves, gowns, masks, and goggles.

6. Feeding and Hydration Assistance: Candidates are evaluated on their ability to assist patients with feeding and drinking while preserving their autonomy and ensuring proper nutrition and hydration.

7. Positioning and Turning Patients: This skill evaluates candidates' proficiency in safely and effectively repositioning and turning patients to enhance their comfort, prevent pressure ulcers, and maintain proper body alignment.

The CNA exam comprises a written (or oral) examination and a skills evaluation. These components assess candidates' knowledge and practical skills in various aspects of nursing assistant responsibilities. To excel in the exam, candidates should prepare thoroughly, demonstrating a comprehensive understanding of nursing concepts, effective communication, and the ability to provide safe and compassionate care to patients.

PRACTICE TEST

CNA Roles, Roles of Others, and Teamwork

1. Question: What is the primary role of a Certified Nursing Assistant (CNA) in a healthcare team?
A) Diagnosing illnesses
B) Prescribing medication
C) Providing primary patient care and assistance
D) Conducting major surgeries

2. Question: Who creates a patient's overall care plan in a healthcare setting?
A) Certified Nursing Assistant
B) Registered Nurse
C) Physical Therapist
D) Patient's family member

3. Question: In a healthcare team, who is primarily responsible for administering medication to patients?
A) Nursing Assistant
B) Pharmacist
C) Licensed Practical Nurse (LPN) or Registered Nurse (RN)
D) Physical Therapist

4. Question: What is the most appropriate action for a CNA when they notice a change in a patient's condition?
A) Immediately tell the patient's family
B) Change the patient's medication
C) Document the change and report it to a nurse
D) Ignore the change, as it is not part of the CNA's responsibilities

5. Question: When working in a team, a CNA is expected to:
A) Take over the responsibilities of a Registered Nurse
B) Work independently without consulting anyone
C) Collaborate and communicate effectively with other team members
D) Make critical decisions about patient care

6. Question: A CNA should understand the scope of their practice. Which of the following is NOT within a CNA's scope of practice?
A) Assisting patients with mobility
B) Providing emotional support to patients
C) Prescribing medication
D) Monitoring vital signs

7. Question: In terms of teamwork, a CNA's role often includes:
A) Supervising other CNAs
B) Collaborating with physical therapists to assist in patient mobility
C) Leading healthcare team meetings
D) Performing major surgical procedures

8. Question: If a CNA encounters a situation that conflicts with their ethical or moral beliefs, they should:
A) Refuse to care for the patient
B) Discuss the situation with their supervisor or a nurse
C) Ignore their feelings and continue with the task
D) Ask another CNA to deal with the situation

9. Question: What is an essential skill for a CNA when participating in a multidisciplinary healthcare team?
A) Advanced surgical skills
B) Effective communication
C) Ability to prescribe treatments
D) Experience in medical billing

10. Question: A CNA notices that a patient's room is not clean. What should they do?
A) Clean the room themselves, regardless of other responsibilities
B) Ignore it, as it is not their job
C) Report the issue to the housekeeping department
D) Complain to the patient about the staff

Legal and Ethical Aspects of the CNA Role

1. Question: A CNA overhears a colleague discussing a patient's private health information with a non-medical staff member. What is the most appropriate action for the CNA to take?
A) Join the conversation and share their opinion
B) Report the incident to a supervisor or the compliance department
C) Ignore it, as it is not their responsibility
D) Share the information with other patients

2. Question: Which of the following actions is considered a violation of a patient's rights?
A) Providing care with respect and dignity
B) Refusing to allow a patient to voice complaints
C) Encouraging a patient to express their preferences
D) Respecting a patient's cultural and religious beliefs

3. Question: When obtaining informed consent for a procedure, whose responsibility is to ensure the patient understands and agrees to it?
A) Certified Nursing Assistant
B) Registered Nurse or Physician
C) Family member of the patient
D) Hospital administrator

4. Question: If a patient expresses a desire to create an advance directive, what should a CNA do?
A) Draft the advance directive for the patient
B) Ignore the request as it is not within their scope
C) Inform the nurse or a responsible healthcare professional
D) Advise the patient on what decisions to make

5. Question: What is the best practice for a CNA when documenting care provided to a patient?
A) Writing notes at the end of the shift for all patients together
B) Documenting care accurately and promptly after providing it
C) Asking a colleague to document on their behalf
D) Exaggerating the care provided for better impressions

6. Question: What should CNAs do if assigned a task outside their scope of practice?
A) Attempt the task to the best of their ability
B) Refuse to work until given appropriate tasks
C) Delegate the task to another CNA
D) Discuss the situation with a supervisor or nurse

7. Question: A patient in a long-term care facility gifts a valuable item to their CNA. What should the CNA do?
A) Accept the gift to avoid offending the patient
B) Politely decline and explain the policy on gifts
C) Accept the gift and report it to a supervisor
D) Ask the patient for a monetary gift instead

8. Question: When can a CNA access a patient's medical record be acceptable?
A) When the CNA is curious about the patient's diagnosis
B) Only when it is relevant to the care they are providing
C) When other staff members are discussing the patient
D) To compare with another patient's condition

9. Question: If a CNA witnesses abuse or neglect in the healthcare setting, they should:
A) Confront the abuser directly
B) Report the incident immediately to a supervisor or appropriate authority
C) Discuss the situation with the patient first
D) Wait to see if it happens again before reporting

10. Question: A CNA is asked to witness a patient signing a consent form. What should the CNA ensure before seeing the signature?
A) That the patient has been given all the necessary information about the procedure
B) That the CNA agrees with the procedure
C) That the nurse properly fills out the form
D) That the patient's family members agree with the decision

Priorities and Priority Setting

1. Question: If a CNA cares for multiple patients, which situation should they address first?
A) A patient who is due for a routine medication
B) A patient who is feeling lonely and wants to talk
C) A patient who has fallen and may be injured
D) A patient who needs help with feeding

2. Question: How should CNAs prioritize tasks if they are assigned to assist with a bathing routine for one patient and feeding another who cannot feed themselves?
A) Start with the task they find easiest
B) Assist the patient with feeding first, then proceed to the bathing routine
C) Ask a colleague to do one of the tasks
D) Do both tasks simultaneously

3. Question: What should a CNA do first when beginning their shift?
A) Take a break to prepare for the shift
B) Check social media for any updates from colleagues
C) Review the care plans and needs of assigned patients
D) Start with the most straightforward tasks to ease into the shift

4. Question: A CNA is scheduled to assist two patients simultaneously: one needs help with a bath, and the other has a physical therapy appointment. What should the CNA do?
A) Assist with the bath first, as it is more relaxing for the patient
B) Help the patient get to their physical therapy appointment on time
C) Ask the patients to decide
D) Cancel the physical therapy appointment

5. Question: When prioritizing care, what should a CNA do if unsure about the urgency of a patient's needs?
A) Guess and act on their intuition
B) Ask the patient what they should do first
C) Seek guidance from a registered nurse or supervisor
D) Choose the task that is closest to their current location

6. Question: If a CNA runs behind schedule, what is the best approach to managing their remaining tasks?
A) Rush through each task to finish on time
B) Skip less critical tasks
C) Prioritize critical patient needs and communicate delays to a nurse or supervisor
D) Leave the remaining tasks for the next shift

7. Question: A patient requires immediate assistance after a medical procedure, but another patient asks for help with a non-urgent task. How should the CNA prioritize these tasks?
A) Help the patient with the non-urgent task first to quickly finish it
B) Attend to the patient who requires immediate assistance after the medical procedure
C) Ask another CNA to handle one of the tasks
D) Alternate between both patients

8. Question: In an emergency on the ward, what should be the CNA's priority?
A) Assisting with the emergency as directed by medical staff
B) Continuing with their routine tasks
C) Evacuating themselves from the ward
D) Informing patient families about the emergency

9. Question: How should a CNA handle a situation where two patients need assistance simultaneously and the tasks are equally important?
A) Assist the patient they like more
B) Use a first-come, first-served approach
C) Seek assistance from other team members to manage both tasks simultaneously
D) Choose randomly

10. Question: What is the best practice for CNAs when assigned a new task while already engaged in another critical study?
A) Immediately switch to the new task
B) Finish the current task quickly, regardless of quality
C) Assess the urgency of the new task and prioritize accordingly
D) Ignore the new task until the current one is completed

Acceptable and Unacceptable Abbreviations

1. Question: Which of the following abbreviations is acceptable in medical documentation?
A) U (for unit)
B) QOD (every other day)
C) BP (for blood pressure)
D) IU (for international unit)

2. Question: When documenting medication dosage, which abbreviation should be avoided?
A) mg (for milligrams)
B) mcg (for micrograms)
C) HS (for at bedtime)
D) PO (for by mouth)

3. Question: What does the abbreviation 'PRN' stand for, and when is it used?
A) Every morning; used for daily routines
B) After meals; used for post-meal activities
C) As needed; used for medications or treatments
D) Before meals; used for pre-meal medications

4. Question: Which abbreviation should be used cautiously due to its potential for being misread?
A) IV (for intravenous)
B) BID (for twice a day)
C) QID (for four times a day)
D) QD (for every day)

5. Question: The abbreviation 'NPO' is used in medical settings. What does it mean?
A) New patient orientation
B) Nothing by mouth
C) Normal post-operative
D) Nightly pain observation

6. Question: Which abbreviations are safe and acceptable for medical documentation?
A) QHS (for every night at bedtime)
B) D/C (for discharge or discontinue)
C) TID (for three times a day)
D) OD (for right eye)

7. Question: What is the appropriate abbreviation for 'before meals'?
A) AC
B) PC
C) BID
D) HS

8. Question: In a medical context, the abbreviation 'SOB' stands for:
A) Shortness of breath
B) Start of business
C) Status on backorder
D) Saturated oxygen binding

9. Question: The abbreviation 'IM' is frequently used in medical settings. What does it represent?
A) Internal medicine
B) Intramuscular
C) Immediate message
D) Intra-membrane

10. Question: Which abbreviation is discouraged in medical records due to potential misinterpretation?
A) BPM (beats per minute)
B) EKG (electrocardiogram)
C) O2 (oxygen)
D) BT (bedtime)

Observation, Reporting, and Abbreviations

1. Question: When observing a patient, a CNA notices a sudden change in skin color. What is the most appropriate action?
A) Wait to see if it changes back
B) Report the observation to a nurse immediately
C) Document the change at the end of the shift
D) Advise the patient to rest more

2. Question: A CNA hears a patient repeatedly coughing during the night. What should they do first?
A) Provide cough syrup to the patient
B) Document the observation in the patient's chart
C) Ignore it, as it is a common occurrence
D) Check on the patient and then report to a nurse

3. Question: What does the ADL abbreviation mean regarding CNA duties?
A) Advanced directive list
B) Activities of daily living
C) Afternoon duty log
D) Authorized drug list

4. Question: What is the best course of action when a CNA notices a patient is not eating their meals?
A) Encourage the patient to eat more
B) Report the observation to a nurse
C) Change the patient's diet without consulting
D) Document the issue but take no further action

5. Question: If a CNA observes that a patient's wound is not healing as expected, what should they do?
A) Apply a different medication to the wound
B) Wait for the next doctor's visit to mention it
C) Report the observation to a nurse immediately
D) Try a home remedy

6. Question: What does the abbreviation 'BID' mean in medical terms?
A) Before infectious diseases
B) Twice a day
C) Brought in dead
D) Before initial diagnosis

7. Question: A CNA observes a patient exhibiting new signs of confusion and disorientation. What should be the first action?
A) Reorient the patient to the time and place
B) Report the changes to a nurse
C) Assume it's a temporary issue and monitor
D) Inform the patient's family members

8. Question: When documenting in a patient's chart, what should a CNA do if they make an error?
A) Erase the error and write over it
B) Use correction fluid to cover it
C) Draw a single line through the error, initial it, and write the correction
D) Leave the error uncorrected

9. Question: The abbreviation 'PR' in medical documentation usually stands for:
A) Pulse rate
B) Per rectum
C) Previous record
D) Patient referral

10. Question: What is the most appropriate action for a CNA if they observe a patient having difficulty breathing?
A) Wait a few minutes to see if it improves
B) Give the patient a glass of water
C) Report the observation to a nurse immediately
D) Provide reassurance to the patient only

Safety and Managing Behavior

1. Question: What should a CNA do first if they find a patient on the floor?
A) Immediately lift the patient back into bed
B) Call for help and assess the patient for any injuries
C) Leave the patient to find a nurse
D) Take a break as the situation is too stressful

2. Question: How should a CNA respond to a patient who is behaving aggressively?
A) Respond with equal aggression
B) Ignore the behavior and continue working
C) Try to reason and argue with the patient
D) Maintain a safe distance and inform a nurse or supervisor

3. Question: What is the most effective way for a CNA to prevent the spread of infection?
A) Wearing gloves at all times
B) Regular hand washing and using personal protective equipment (PPE) appropriately
C) Taking antibiotics regularly
D) Limiting contact with patients

4. Question: A patient with dementia repeatedly tries to leave the unit. What should a CNA do?
A) Restrain the patient physically
B) Distract and redirect the patient and inform the nursing staff
C) Lock the patient in their room
D) Scold the patient for trying to leave

5. Question: What is the primary reason for using a gait belt when assisting patients with mobility?
A) To control the patient's movements
B) For the CNA's convenience
C) To provide stability and safety for the patient
D) To track the patient's walking distance

6. Question: If a patient refuses a planned activity, what is the best response by the CNA?
A) Force the patient to participate
B) Report the refusal to a nurse and respect the patient's decision
C) Ignore the refusal and leave the patient alone
D) Bribe the patient to participate

7. Question: How should a CNA respond to a verbally abusive patient?
A) Engage in the verbal abuse
B) Politely excuse themselves and report the behavior to a supervisor
C) Ignore the abuse and continue working
D) Argue back to defend themselves

8. Question: What is the most crucial action when a fire alarm goes off in a healthcare facility?
A) Immediately evacuate all patients by yourself
B) Panic and run to find an exit
C) Follow the facility's fire safety and evacuation protocols
D) Hide in a safe place until the alarm stops

9. Question: What should a CNA do if unsure how to operate medical equipment?
A) Try to use it based on instinct
B) Ask a colleague who is also unsure
C) Avoid using it altogether
D) Seek guidance from a nurse or trained staff member

10. Question: When a patient is at risk of falling, what is an appropriate measure?
A) Use physical restraints as a precaution
B) Place a bed alarm on the patient's bed
C) Leave the patient unattended to encourage independence
D) Increase the sedation of the patient

Disasters and Emergencies

1. Question: What is the first action a CNA should take in the event of an earthquake while working in a healthcare facility?
A) Immediately evacuate all patients
B) Stay calm and follow the facility's earthquake safety procedures
C) Hide under a desk or bed
D) Call family members to inform them about the earthquake

2. Question: During a fire emergency, what is the priority for a CNA?
A) To save personal belongings
B) To ensure the safety and evacuation of patients, if possible
C) To extinguish the fire
D) To document the event for records

3. Question: If a CNA discovers a small, contained fire in a patient's room, what should they do first?
A) Try to put it out with water
B) Close the door to contain the fire and activate the fire alarm
C) Evacuate the entire floor
D) Call the fire department
4. Question: How should a CNA respond to a tornado warning while on duty?
A) Open all windows to equalize pressure
B) Continue with regular duties until further notice
C) Move patients to designated safe areas according to the facility's tornado response plan
D) Evacuate the building

5. Question: In the event of a power outage in a healthcare facility, what is the primary concern for a CNA?
A) Checking if the television and other entertainment systems are working
B) Ensuring all electronic devices are charged
C) Ensuring patient safety and checking on life-support equipment
D) Finding a flashlight to continue with routine tasks

6. Question: What is the most appropriate action for a CNA during a facility lockdown?
A) Attempt to leave the facility immediately
B) Call external authorities to ask for advice
C) Follow the facility's lockdown procedures and ensure patient safety
D) Use social media to update about the situation

7. Question: How should a CNA prepare for a potential healthcare facility evacuation?
A) Pack personal items to take with them
B) Familiarize themselves with the evacuation routes and procedures
C) Decide which patients to evacuate first based on personal preference
D) Wait for instructions at the time of evacuation

8. Question: In case of a hazardous material spill in the facility, what should a CNA do?
A) Clean it up immediately to prevent panic
B) Evacuate the patients from the facility
C) Notify the appropriate personnel and follow the facility's hazardous material protocol
D) Take a picture of the spill for the facility's records

9. Question: What should a CNA do if a patient becomes violent during a stressful emergency?
A) Attempt to restrain the patient alone physically
B) Try to calm the patient and seek help from a nurse or security
C) Leave the patient alone until they calm down
D) Use verbal threats to control the patient

10. Question: What is the best course of action if a CNA needs clarification on the correct procedure during an emergency?
A) Guess and proceed with what seems best
B) Wait and hope someone else takes charge
C) Ask a colleague for their opinion
D) Seek immediate clarification from a supervisor or follow the facility's emergency protocols

Personal Care Skills

1. Question: What is the most crucial aspect to remember when assisting a patient with bathing?
A) Completing the bath as quickly as possible
B) Ensuring the patient's privacy and comfort
C) Using as much soap and water as possible
D) Bathing the patient without their consent to save time

2. Question: When helping a patient to dress, what should a CNA prioritize?
A) Choosing clothes that the CNA likes
B) Allowing the patient to choose their attire, if able
C) Dressing the patient quickly, regardless of their preferences
D) Choosing clothes that are easy for the CNA to put on the patient

3. Question: In assisting with oral hygiene, what should a CNA do if a patient has dentures?
A) Avoid cleaning the dentures as they can be fragile
B) Clean the dentures daily along with the patient's natural teeth
C) Leave the dentures out for an extended period
D) Use hot water for cleaning the dentures

4. Question: How should a CNA assist a patient with mobility issues in transferring from a bed to a wheelchair?
A) By lifting the patient quickly and efficiently
B) Using proper body mechanics and, if necessary, a transfer/gait belt
C) By having the patient transfer themselves, regardless of their ability
D) Calling another patient to assist

5. Question: What is a crucial consideration when providing incontinence care to a patient?
A) Completing the task as rapidly as possible
B) Ensuring patient privacy and dignity throughout the process
C) Using cold water to clean the patient
D) Limiting fluid intake to reduce incontinence

6. Question: What should a CNA do when feeding a patient who has difficulty swallowing?
A) Feed them quickly to avoid taking too much time
B) Encourage the patient to take large bites to expedite feeding
C) Allow the patient to lie flat to make it easier to swallow
D) Assist the patient in sitting upright and offer small bites

7. Question: What is an appropriate action for a CNA when assisting a patient with grooming?
A) Ignore the patient's preferences to make grooming faster
B) Involve the patient in decisions about their grooming
C) Choose a hairstyle that is easiest for the CNA to manage
D) Use any products available, regardless of the patient's skin type

8. Question: How should a CNA approach nail care for a diabetic patient?
A) Avoid it altogether, as it's too risky
B) Cut the nails as short as possible
C) File the nails instead of cutting and check for any signs of infection
D) Soak the feet in hot water before nail care

9. Question: What is a crucial aspect a CNA should consider when providing hair care?
A) Washing the hair daily, regardless of the patient's condition
B) Brushing or combing the hair gently to prevent tangles and discomfort
C) Styling the hair in complex ways to improve the patient's mood
D) Ignoring the patient's hair type and texture

10. Question: What is the correct approach for a CNA when assisting a patient with ambulation?
A) Encourage fast walking to improve strength
B) Let the patient walk alone for independence
C) Provide support as needed and stay close to assist
D) Use a wheelchair at all times to prevent falls

ANSWER KEY

CNA Roles, Roles of Others, and Teamwork

1. **Answer: C) Providing primary patient care and assistance**
   Explanation: CNAs are trained to assist patients with primary care needs, such as bathing, dressing, and feeding, rather than diagnosing or treating illnesses.
2. **Answer: B) Registered Nurse**
   Explanation: Registered Nurses (RNs) typically oversee the creation and implementing of a patient's care plan, although they work collaboratively with the entire healthcare team.
3. **Answer: C) Licensed Practical Nurse (LPN) or Registered Nurse (RN)**
   Explanation: LPNs and RNs are generally responsible for administering medication, which requires professional nursing licensure.
4. **Answer: C) Document the change and report it to a nurse**
   Explanation: CNAs should document any changes in a patient's condition and report them to a nurse for further assessment and action.
5. **Answer: C) Collaborate and communicate effectively with other team members**
   Explanation: Effective teamwork in healthcare requires CNAs to collaborate and communicate with other team members to ensure coordinated and comprehensive patient care.
6. **Answer: C) Prescribing medication**
   Explanation: Prescribing medication is beyond the scope of practice for a CNA and is reserved for licensed medical professionals such as physicians and nurse practitioners.
7. **Answer: B) Collaborating with physical therapists to assist in patient mobility**
   Explanation: CNAs often collaborate with physical therapists and other healthcare professionals to assist in the mobility and rehabilitation of patients.
8. **Answer: B) Discuss the situation with their supervisor or a nurse**
   Explanation: CNAs should discuss ethical or moral conflicts with their supervisor or a nurse to find an appropriate solution while maintaining professional conduct.
9. **Answer: B) Effective communication**
   Explanation: Effective communication is crucial for CNAs to relay information accurately and work collaboratively within a multidisciplinary healthcare team.
10. **Answer: C) Report the issue to the housekeeping department**
    Explanation: CNAs should report such matters to the appropriate department (like housekeeping) to ensure the patient's safe and clean environment.

Legal and Ethical Aspects of the CNA Role

1. **Answer: B) Report the incident to a supervisor or the compliance department**
   Explanation: CNAs must maintain patient confidentiality and report any breaches, such as discussing private health information with unauthorized personnel, to uphold legal and ethical standards.
2. **Answer: B) Refusing to allow a patient to voice complaints**
   Explanation: Patients have the right to voice complaints about their care. Preventing them from doing so violates their rights and is unethical.
3. **Answer: B) Registered Nurse or Physician**
   Explanation: Obtaining informed consent is typically the RN or physician's responsibility to perform or oversee the procedure. It is beyond the scope of practice for a CNA.
4. **Answer: C) Inform the nurse or a responsible healthcare professional**
   Explanation: CNAs should report the patient's request to a nurse or healthcare professional who can provide appropriate assistance, as creating an advance directive is beyond the CNA's scope.
5. **Answer: B) Documenting care accurately and promptly after providing it**
   Explanation: Accurate and timely documentation is crucial in healthcare for maintaining legal and ethical standards of care.

6. **Answer: D) Discuss the situation with a supervisor or nurse**
   Explanation: CNAs should communicate with their supervisor or a nurse when asked to perform tasks outside their scope to ensure safe and legal care.
7. **Answer: B) Politely decline and explain the policy on gifts**
   Explanation: CNAs should adhere to professional boundaries and ethical guidelines, which often include declining gifts, especially of significant value, to avoid conflicts of interest.
8. **Answer: B) Only when it is relevant to the care they are providing**
   Explanation: CNAs should access patient records only for reasons pertinent to their care, respecting privacy and confidentiality laws.
9. **Answer: B) Report the incident immediately to a supervisor or appropriate authority**
   Explanation: CNAs have a legal and ethical obligation to promptly report any observed abuse or neglect to a supervisor or appropriate authority.
10. **Answer: A) That the patient has been given all the necessary information about the procedure**
    Explanation: While witnessing a consent form, the CNA should ensure that the patient is informed and consenting voluntarily, although verifying the details of the information is usually beyond the CNA's role.

Priorities and Priority Setting

1. **Answer: C) A patient who has fallen and may be injured**
   Explanation: Addressing immediate safety concerns, like a patient who has lost, is a top priority to prevent harm.
2. **Answer: B) Assist the patient with feeding first, then proceed to the bathing routine**
   Explanation: Basic needs like feeding should be prioritized over routine tasks like bathing, especially when patients cannot feed themselves.
3. **Answer: C) Review the care plans and needs of assigned patients**
   Explanation: Reviewing care plans and patient needs at the start of a shift helps CNAs prioritize tasks and provide adequate care.
4. **Answer: B) Help the patient get to their physical therapy appointment on time**
   Explanation: Ensuring patients attend scheduled appointments, especially for therapies, is essential and should be prioritized over routine care tasks.
5. **Answer: C) Seek guidance from a registered nurse or supervisor**
   Explanation: CNAs should consult a nurse or supervisor for advice to ensure patient safety and proper care when prioritizing tasks.
6. **Answer: C) Prioritize critical patient needs and communicate delays to a nurse or supervisor**
   Explanation: Prioritizing urgent needs and communicating with the healthcare team about delays ensures patient safety and continuity of care.
7. **Answer: B) Attend to the patient who requires immediate assistance after the medical procedure**
   Explanation: Immediate medical needs following a procedure should be prioritized over non-urgent tasks to ensure patient safety and proper recovery.
8. **Answer: A) Assisting with the emergency as directed by medical staff**
   Explanation: In an emergency, CNAs should assist as directed by medical staff, prioritizing patient safety and following emergency protocols.
9. **Answer: C) Seek assistance from other team members to manage both tasks simultaneously**
   Explanation: Collaborating with other team members can help manage simultaneous, equally essential tasks efficiently and effectively.
10. **Answer: C) Assess the urgency of the new task and prioritize accordingly**
    Explanation: CNAs should assess the urgency and importance of functions to determine the best order of completion, ensuring patient needs are met effectively.

Acceptable and Unacceptable Abbreviations

1. **Answer: C) BP (for blood pressure)**
   Explanation: 'BP' is a widely recognized and acceptable abbreviation for 'blood pressure.' Abbreviations like 'U,' 'QOD,' and 'IU' are often discouraged due to potential confusion or misinterpretation.

2. **Answer: C) HS (for at bedtime)**
   Explanation: 'HS' can be confused with 'half-strength' or 'hours of sleep,' leading to errors in medication administration. The other abbreviations are standard and acceptable.

3. **Answer: C) As needed; used for medications or treatments**
   Explanation: 'PRN' is an acceptable abbreviation for 'pro re nata,' a Latin phrase meaning 'as needed.' It is commonly used for medications or treatments that are not on a regular schedule but are administered as required.

4. **Answer: D) QD (for every day)**
   Explanation: 'QD' can easily be mistaken for 'QID' (four times a day) if written poorly. It's safer to write 'daily' to avoid confusion.

5. **Answer: B) Nothing by mouth**
   Explanation: 'NPO' stands for 'nil per os,' a Latin term meaning 'nothing by mouth.' It indicates that a patient should not take anything orally, often before surgery or specific medical tests.

6. **Answer: C) TID (for three times a day)**
   Explanation: 'TID' is a standard abbreviation for 'ter in die,' meaning 'three times a day,' and is widely accepted in medical documentation. Other abbreviations like 'QHS,' 'D/C,' and 'OD' can be ambiguous or misunderstood.

7. **Answer: A) AC**
   Explanation: 'AC' stands for 'ante cibum,' Latin for 'before meals'. It is commonly used in the context of medication timing.

8. **Answer: A) Shortness of breath**
   Explanation: In healthcare, 'SOB' is an acceptable abbreviation for 'shortness of breath,' a common symptom in many medical conditions.

9. **Answer: B) Intramuscular**
   Explanation: 'IM' is a standard abbreviation for 'intramuscular,' commonly used for injections directly into a muscle.

10. **Answer: D) BT (bedtime)**
    Explanation: 'BT' can be confused with 'BMT' (bone marrow transplant) or 'BRT' (be right there). Writing out 'bedtime' is safer to ensure clarity in patient care instructions.

Observation, Reporting, and Abbreviations

1. **Answer: B) Report the observation to a nurse immediately**
   Explanation: Sudden changes in a patient's skin color can be significant and should be reported to a nurse immediately for further assessment.

2. **Answer: D) Check on the patient and then report to a nurse**
   Explanation: The CNA should check on the patient for immediate needs or distress and then write the observation to a nurse for further action.

3. **Answer: B) Activities of daily living**
   Explanation: 'ADL' stands for 'activities of daily living,' which refers to daily self-care activities that CNAs often assist patients with.

4. **Answer: B) Report the observation to a nurse**
   Explanation: A change in eating habits can be significant. The CNA should report this observation to a nurse for further evaluation and intervention.

5. **Answer: C) Report the observation to a nurse immediately**
   Explanation: Any concerns about wound healing should be reported to a nurse promptly for appropriate medical assessment and intervention.

6. **Answer: B) Twice a day**
   Explanation: 'BID' is a standard medical abbreviation for 'bis in die,' Latin for 'twice a day.'

7. **Answer: B) Report the changes to a nurse**

Explanation: New signs of confusion and disorientation are potentially serious and should be reported to a nurse immediately for evaluation.

8. **Answer: C) Draw a single line through the error, initial it, and write the correction**
Explanation: The correct way to amend a documentation error is to draw a single line through it, initial it, and then write the accurate information. This maintains the integrity of the record.

9. **Answer: B) Per rectum**
Explanation: In medical terminology, 'PR' is commonly used to denote 'per rectum,' particularly in the context of specific examinations or medication administration routes.

10. **Answer: C) Report the observation to a nurse immediately**
Explanation: Difficulty breathing is a potentially serious symptom that requires immediate attention. The CNA should promptly report this to a nurse for further evaluation and necessary intervention.

Safety and Managing Behavior

1. **Answer: B) Call for help and assess the patient for any injuries**
Explanation: The first action should be to call for help and quickly evaluate the patient for injuries, ensuring their safety before moving them.

2. **Answer: D) Maintain a safe distance and inform a nurse or supervisor**
Explanation: When dealing with aggression, maintaining safety is paramount. The CNA should keep a safe space and report the behavior to a nurse or supervisor for appropriate intervention.

3. **Answer: B) Regular hand washing and using personal protective equipment (PPE) appropriately**
Explanation: Regular hand washing and proper use of PPE are critical practices in preventing the spread of infections in healthcare settings.

4. **Answer: B) Distract and redirect the patient and inform the nursing staff**
Explanation: Distracting and turning the patient's attention is safe and effective. The behavior should also be reported to the nursing staff for further management.

5. **Answer: C) To provide stability and safety for the patient**
Explanation: A gait belt is used to help stabilize and support the patient during transfers and ambulation, enhancing safety.

6. **Answer: B) Report the refusal to a nurse and respect the patient's decision**
Explanation: The CNA should report the refusal to a nurse and respect the patient's right to refuse treatment or activities while ensuring their safety.

7. **Answer: B) Politely excuse themselves and report the behavior to a supervisor**
Explanation: The CNAs should maintain professionalism, remove themselves from the abusive situation, and report the behavior to a supervisor for appropriate action.

8. **Answer: C) Follow the facility's fire safety and evacuation protocols**
Explanation: In the event of a fire alarm, following the facility's established fire safety and evacuation protocols is crucial for the safety of both patients and staff.

9. **Answer: D) Seek guidance from a nurse or trained staff member**
Explanation: If unsure about using medical equipment, the CNA should seek instruction and advice from a nurse or a trained staff member to ensure patient safety and proper equipment usage.

10. **Answer: B) Place a bed alarm on the patient's bed**
Explanation: Using a bed alarm is a non-restrictive measure to alert staff if a patient is at risk of falling attempts to get up, enhancing patient safety.

Disasters and Emergencies

1. **Answer: B) Stay calm and follow the facility's earthquake safety procedures**
   Explanation: In an earthquake, the CNA should remain calm and follow the established earthquake safety procedures of the healthcare facility to ensure their safety and that of the patients.
2. **Answer: B) To ensure the safety and evacuation of patients, if possible**
   Explanation: In a fire emergency, the primary responsibility of a CNA is to ensure the safety and evacuation of patients, following the facility's fire response protocol.
3. **Answer: B) Close the door to contain the fire and activate the fire alarm**
   Explanation: The first step is to have the fire, if possible, and start the fire alarm to alert others, followed by following the facility's fire response procedures.
4. **Answer: C) Move patients to designated safe areas according to the facility's tornado response plan**
   Explanation: During a warning, the CNA should move patients to pre-designated safe areas following the facility's tornado response plan.
5. **Answer: C) Ensuring patient safety and checking on life-support equipment**
   Explanation: In a power outage, the main concern is patient safety, mainly checking on those dependent on electronic life-support equipment.
6. **Answer: C) Follow the facility's lockdown procedures and ensure patient safety**
   Explanation: During a lockdown, the CNA should adhere to the facility's specific lockdown procedures, focusing on ensuring the safety and calmness of patients.
7. **Answer: B) Familiarize themselves with the evacuation routes and procedures**
   Explanation: Being familiar with evacuation routes and procedures is crucial for a CNA to assist in a potential evacuation scenario effectively.
8. **Answer: C) Notify the appropriate personnel and follow the facility's hazardous material protocol**
   Explanation: A CNA should notify the appropriate personnel and follow the established hazardous material protocol of the facility to handle such situations safely, ensuring staff and patient safety.
9. **Answer: B) Try to calm the patient and seek help from a nurse or security**
   Explanation: The CNA should attempt to collect the patient and immediately seek assistance from a nurse or security personnel to manage the situation safely.
10. **Answer: D) Seek immediate clarification from a supervisor or follow the facility's emergency protocols.**
    Explanation: In any emergency where a CNA is unsure, seeking immediate clarification from a supervisor or following the established emergency protocols of the facility ensures that actions are taken based on correct procedures.

Personal Care Skills

1. **Answer: B) Ensuring the patient's privacy and comfort**
   Explanation: While assisting with bathing, it's crucial to maintain the patient's privacy and ensure their comfort, respecting their dignity and preferences.

2. **Answer: B) Allowing the patient to choose their attire, if able**
   Explanation: Encouraging patient independence and respecting their choices, such as selecting clothes, is essential for promoting dignity and autonomy.

3. **Answer: B) Clean the dentures daily along with the patient's natural teeth**
   Explanation: Dentures should be cleaned daily to maintain oral hygiene. It's essential to handle them with care and follow proper cleaning procedures.

4. **Answer: B) Using proper body mechanics and, if necessary, a transfer/gait belt.**
   Explanation: Proper body mechanics and assistive devices like a transfer or gait belt help ensure the patients' and the CNAs' safety during transfers.

5. **Answer: B) Ensuring patient privacy and dignity throughout the process**
   Explanation: Maintaining the patient's privacy and dignity is essential during incontinence care. It's important to be respectful and gentle while providing thorough care.

6. **Answer: D) Assist the patient in sitting upright and offer small bites**
   Explanation: Sitting upright can prevent choking for a patient with difficulty swallowing, and small bites can make eating more accessible and safer.

7. **Answer: B) Involve the patient in decisions about their grooming**
   Explanation: Involving the patient in grooming decisions respects their autonomy and preferences, contributing to their sense of self and well-being.

8. **Answer: C) File the nails instead of cutting and check for any signs of infection**
   Explanation: Diabetic patients are at higher risk of infection and foot complications. Filing instead of cutting reduces the risk of cuts, and it's important to monitor for any signs of infection.

9. **Answer: B) Brushing or combing the hair gently to prevent tangles and discomfort**
   Explanation: Gentle hair care, including brushing or combing to prevent tangles, is essential for patient comfort and scalp health.

10. **Answer: C) Provide support as needed and stay close to assist**
    Explanation: When assisting with ambulation, it's essential to provide appropriate support, stay close to help, and ensure the patient's safety, adjusting the level of assistance based on their ability.

HOSPITAL-ACQUIRED INFECTIONS (HAIS)

Hospital-acquired infections (HAIs), often termed nosocomial infections, refer to infections that patients acquire while receiving medical care in a hospital or another healthcare facility. These infections can occur in any part of the body, including the urinary tract, bloodstream, respiratory system, or surgical sites. Notably, HAIs are not present at the time of admission; instead, they develop during a patient's treatment.

The significance of understanding and preventing HAIs for a Certified Nursing Assistant (CNA) cannot be overstated. These infections can result in prolonged hospital stays, increased healthcare costs, and, in severe cases, may even lead to death. Moreover, many HAIs are preventable, emphasizing the importance of adhering to infection control practices.

Types of HAIs

Catheter-Associated Urinary Tract Infections (CAUTIs): This type of infection occurs when germs enter the urinary system through a catheter. It is one of the most common HAIs in the United States. Proper catheter care, including ensuring it is clean and only in place when necessary, can help reduce the risk of CAUTIs.

Surgical Site Infections (SSIs): SSIs occur in the area of the body where surgery was performed. Depending on the location and depth of the procedure, SSIs can be superficial (involving just the skin) or more serious, impacting organs or implanted material. Proper wound care and maintaining a sterile environment during surgical procedures are essential in preventing SSIs.

Central Line-Associated Bloodstream Infections (CLABSIs): CLABSIs happen when harmful bacteria enter the bloodstream through a central line, a tube that doctors place near the heart to administer medication or collect blood. Maintaining cleanliness while inserting the central line and ensuring that it remains uncontaminated during its use is pivotal in reducing the chances of a CLABSI.

Ventilator-Associated Pneumonia (VAP): VAP is a lung infection that develops in people who are on mechanical ventilation through endotracheal intubation or tracheostomy. It's vital for healthcare providers to maintain oral hygiene for intubated patients and to ensure that the ventilator's equipment is sterile to mitigate the risk of VAP.

Clostridium difficile Infections: Often abbreviated as C. diff, this bacterium can cause symptoms ranging from diarrhea to life-threatening colon inflammation. The infection typically occurs after the use of antibiotic medications. Hand hygiene, especially with soap and water, plays a crucial role in preventing the spread of C. diff, as alcohol-based hand sanitizers may not effectively eliminate it.

For a CNA, understanding HAIs and the means to prevent them is paramount. Each HAI type has its unique set of risk factors and prevention strategies. Adhering to best practices in cleanliness, patient care, and medical procedures can significantly reduce the prevalence of these infections, ensuring a safer healthcare environment for all.

How Hospital-Acquired Infections (HAIs) Can Happen?

Hospital-acquired infections (HAIs) pose significant challenges to the healthcare system, not only due to their impact on patient health but also the economic burden they present. For Certified Nursing Assistants (CNAs) and other healthcare professionals, it's crucial to understand how these infections can occur to develop effective prevention strategies. Here's an in-depth look at how HAIs can happen:

Breakdown in Sterile Technique: A significant portion of HAIs can be traced back to a breakdown in sterile techniques. This includes not cleaning hands properly before a procedure, not wearing gloves or changing them as needed, and not ensuring that the environment and tools are sterile. Even a minor lapse can introduce pathogens into sensitive areas.

Improper Use or Maintenance of Medical Devices: Devices like catheters, ventilators, and central lines, if not used or maintained correctly, can be conduits for pathogens. For example, a urinary catheter that isn't inserted using a sterile technique or that remains in place longer than necessary raises the risk of CAUTIs.

Transmission Between Healthcare Workers and Patients: Healthcare workers, due to the nature of their jobs, interact with multiple patients daily. If they don't adhere to proper hand hygiene between patients, they can unwittingly transfer pathogens from one patient to another.

Patient's Flora Becoming Pathogenic: Not all infections come from external sources. Sometimes, a patient's microbial flora, which usually doesn't cause harm, can become pathogenic. This is particularly true when the patient's immune system is compromised or when there's an imbalance caused, for example, by broad-spectrum antibiotics. Such an imbalance can lead to infections like C. difficile.

Overuse or Misuse of Antibiotics: Excessive or inappropriate use of antibiotics can lead to antibiotic resistance, where bacteria evolve to become impervious to the antibiotics used to treat them. This can result in hard-to-treat infections and can significantly raise the risk of HAIs.

Cross-Contamination from Surfaces and Equipment: Pathogens can survive on various surfaces for extended periods, ranging from hours to days. Hospital equipment, bed linens, doorknobs, and even electronic devices can harbor these germs. If they aren't cleaned and disinfected regularly, they can become a source of HAIs.

Airborne Transmission: Some pathogens, like those causing tuberculosis, can be airborne. Inadequate ventilation, improper handling of respiratory equipment, or failure to isolate patients with airborne diseases can lead to the spread of such infections.

Compromised Patient Immunity: Patients in hospitals, especially those in intensive care units or undergoing surgeries, often have weakened immune systems, either from their underlying illness or the treatments they're undergoing. A compromised immune system is less capable of fending off infections, making patients more susceptible to HAIs.

Invasive Procedures: Any procedure that breaks the skin or mucous membranes provides an opportunity for pathogens to enter. Surgeries, injections, and the insertion of medical devices can all introduce germs into the body if not done with utmost care.

Food and Water in Healthcare Settings: If not stored, handled, or prepared correctly, food and water can become sources of infections. It's crucial to ensure that hospital food service operations adhere to the highest standards of cleanliness.

Understanding the myriad ways HAIs can occur is the first step in preventing them. For healthcare professionals, vigilance, continued education, and strict adherence to infection control protocols are essential. The fight against HAIs is ongoing, and every individual in a healthcare setting plays a vital role in this battle.

Catheter-Associated Urinary Tract Infections (CAUTIs)

Catheter-associated urinary Tract Infections (CAUTIs) represent one of the most common healthcare-associated infections in American hospitals. While any patient with a urinary catheter can develop a CAUTI, understanding the causes and implementing preventive measures can drastically reduce the incidence. Let's delve into what CAUTIs are, how they develop, and how they can be avoided.

Understanding CAUTIs: A urinary catheter is a flexible tube that's inserted into the bladder to drain urine. When this catheter becomes a conduit for bacteria to enter the bladder, it can lead to a CAUTI. Notably, the longer a catheter remains in place, the higher the risk of infection, which can then spread to the kidneys or the bloodstream.

Symptoms of CAUTIs: Even though catheterized patients may not exhibit the typical symptoms of a urinary tract infection (UTI) due to the catheter's presence, some signs might indicate a CAUTI:

- Cloudy or bloody urine.
- Foul or strong urine odor.
- Fever or chills.
- Increased confusion or agitation in older adults.
- Discomfort, pain, or burning around the catheter site or in the lower abdomen.

Causes of CAUTIs

- **Introduction of Bacteria at Insertion:** If not properly cleaned, the area around the urethra can introduce bacteria during catheter insertion.
- **Bacteria Traveling up the Catheter:** Over time, bacteria can travel up the external surface of the catheter and into the bladder.
- **Contaminated Urine Collection System:** If the urine collection bag gets contaminated, bacteria can ascend into the bladder.
- **Prolonged Catheter Use:** The longer a catheter is in place, the higher the risk of bacterial colonization and infection.

Tips to Avoid CAUTIs

- **Only Use When Necessary:** Catheters should only be used when there's a valid medical reason and should be removed as soon as they're no longer needed.
- **Sterile Insertion:** Always ensure that the catheter is inserted using a sterile technique. This includes cleaning the urethral area thoroughly, using sterile gloves, and employing a single-use, sterile catheter kit.
- **Regular Cleaning:** The area around the catheter should be cleaned daily and after every bowel movement. This reduces the risk of bacteria traveling up the catheter.
- **Maintain a Closed System:** The catheter and its bag should be kept in a closed system. This means connections should only be opened if necessary (e.g., when changing the bag).
- **Proper Bag Position:** Keep the urine collection bag below the level of the bladder. This prevents the backflow of urine, which can introduce bacteria into the bladder.
- **Avoid Blockages:** Ensure the catheter doesn't become twisted or kinked, allowing urine to flow freely. Stagnant urine can become a breeding ground for bacteria.
- **Regularly Empty the Bag:** Don't allow the urine collection bag to get too full. It should be emptied at least every 8 hours, or sooner if full.
- **Hydration:** Encourage the patient to drink plenty of fluids unless medically contraindicated. This helps in flushing bacteria from the urinary system.
- **Staff Education:** Healthcare staff should be regularly trained and updated on best practices for catheter care to prevent CAUTIs.
- **Monitor for Symptoms:** Stay vigilant for signs of an infection. Early detection and treatment can prevent complications.

CAUTIs, while common, are largely preventable. The key lies in understanding the potential routes of infection and maintaining rigorous hygiene and care standards. As healthcare professionals, including

Certified Nursing Assistants, we play a pivotal role in ensuring patient safety and well-being. By implementing and adhering to best practices in catheter care, we can significantly reduce the risk of CAUTIs and improve patient outcomes. Whether you're inserting a catheter, maintaining it, or educating a patient on its care, remember that attention to detail can make all the difference.

Surgical Site Infections (SSIs)

Surgical Site Infections (SSIs) are among the most frequent and consequential complications following surgeries in American healthcare settings. By definition, an SSI occurs at the site of a surgical incision within 30 days of the procedure or one year if an implant is placed. An understanding of the causes and preventive measures of SSIs is paramount for healthcare professionals aiming to offer the highest standard of patient care.

Understanding SSIs: Surgical Site Infections can range from superficial infections affecting the skin alone to more severe ones involving tissues under the skin, organs, or implanted materials. The impact of SSIs extends beyond physical health; it includes prolonged hospital stays, increased healthcare costs, and, in some cases, long-term disabilities or even death.

Symptoms of SSIs: While symptoms might vary depending on the severity of the infection, common indicators include:

- Redness and warmth at the incision site.
- Swelling around the surgical area.
- Purulent discharge from the incision.
- Persistent pain or tenderness at the surgical site.
- Fever or chills.

Factors Contributing to SSIs: Several factors can increase the likelihood of an SSI:

- **Type of Surgery:** Some surgeries inherently carry a higher risk of SSIs due to their complexity or the area being operated on.
- **Duration of Surgery:** Longer surgical procedures might heighten the risk of infection.
- **Health Status:** Patients with weakened immune systems, diabetes, or obesity are at a higher risk.
- **Sterile Environment:** Any breach in the sterile environment of the operating room can introduce pathogens.

Tips to Avoid SSIs

Preoperative Measures

- **Antibiotic Prophylaxis:** Administering antibiotics before surgery, especially in high-risk procedures, can significantly reduce the risk of SSIs.
- **Skin Preparation:** Properly preparing and disinfecting the skin before incisions are made is crucial. This often involves cleaning the area with antiseptic agents.
- **Maintain Glycemic Control:** For diabetic patients, maintaining blood sugar levels within a normal range around the time of surgery can reduce the risk of SSIs.

Intraoperative Measures

- **Maintain a Sterile Environment:** Ensure that all surgical instruments are sterilized and the operating room adheres to the highest cleanliness standards.
- **Minimize Operating Time:** While it's not always possible, reducing the time a patient spends in surgery can decrease SSI risk.
- **Limit Traffic:** The number of people entering and leaving the operating room should be kept to a minimum during surgery to reduce the introduction of pathogens.

Postoperative Measures

- **Incision Care:** The surgical site should be regularly inspected for signs of infection. It should be kept clean and dry, and any dressings should be changed using a sterile technique.
- **Hand Hygiene:** Ensure that anyone who touches the surgical site, including the patient, has thoroughly cleaned their hands.
- **Educate Patients:** Before discharge, patients should be educated on how to care for their wounds, signs of infections, and when to seek medical advice.

General Tips

- **Proper Nutrition:** A well-nourished body can better resist infection. Ensure patients receive adequate nutrition before and after surgery.
- **Avoid Shaving Surgical Sites:** If hair needs to be removed, it's better to clip than to shave, as shaving can cause tiny nicks in the skin, providing an entry point for bacteria.
- **Regular Training:** Healthcare staff should be routinely updated on best practices for preventing SSIs. This includes surgeons, nurses, and even housekeeping staff responsible for operating room cleanliness.

The prevention of Surgical Site Infections demands a multidisciplinary approach and unwavering diligence. From the initial decision to operate to the postoperative care, every step has the potential to influence the outcome concerning SSIs. By staying informed and implementing best practices, healthcare professionals can play a pivotal role in minimizing the incidence and impact of these infections, ensuring that patients have the best chance for uncomplicated recoveries. In the complex realm of surgical care, details matter, and even the most uncomplicated measures can make a profound difference.

Central Line-Associated Bloodstream Infections (CLABSIs)

Central Line-Associated Bloodstream Infections (CLABSIs) represent a severe challenge in healthcare, often resulting in significant morbidity, extended hospital stays, increased cost of care, and even mortality. As the name suggests, a CLABSI is a bloodstream infection that occurs when bacteria or viruses enter the bloodstream through a central line—a widely used medical tool.

Understanding CLABSIs: A central line, often referred to as a central catheter, is a long, flexible tube placed in a large vein, typically in the neck, chest, arm, or groin. Its primary purpose is to deliver medications fluids, or to collect blood samples. Unlike the standard IV, which is inserted into veins of the hand or arm, a central line reaches more prominent veins near the heart, providing a more direct route to the bloodstream. This positioning, while beneficial, also carries an inherent risk, providing an avenue for pathogens to enter the bloodstream if not appropriately managed.

Symptoms of CLABSIs: While symptoms might differ depending on the patient and the infecting organism, common signs include:

- Fever and chills without an apparent source.
- Redness, warmth, or tenderness at or near the catheter site.
- Drainage from the skin around the central line.
- Elevated white blood cell count.

Factors Contributing to CLABSIs: Some primary causes and risk factors include:

- **Duration of Central Line Use:** The longer a central line remains in place, the higher the risk of infection.
- **Improper Insertion:** If an aseptic technique is not strictly adhered to during insertion, pathogens can be introduced.
- **Inadequate Care:** Regular cleaning and maintenance of the central line and its entry point is necessary for bacteria to colonize the line.
- **Underlying Medical Conditions:** Patients with weakened immune systems or certain chronic illnesses face a heightened risk.

Tips to Avoid CLABSIs

Aseptic Technique for Insertion

- Ensure that the insertion site is cleaned and disinfected meticulously using appropriate antiseptics.
- Use sterile barriers, such as gloves, gowns, caps, and masks, during the procedure.
- Opt for sites less prone to infection. For instance, the subclavian site is often preferred over the femoral or jugular sites when feasible.

Regular Maintenance and Care:

- Check dressings daily to ensure they're clean, dry, and securely in place. Any wet, dirty, or loose dressings should be changed immediately.
- Use a sterile technique when changing dressings, typically employing chlorhexidine-alcohol for skin disinfection.
- Limit the number of manipulations of the catheter and access ports.

Staff Education and Training

- Continuous training for all healthcare workers involved in the insertion and care of central lines is paramount. This includes doctors, nurses, and any other relevant staff.
- Regularly update protocols and guidelines to align with current best practices.

Assess Necessity Daily: Assess the need for the central line daily. If it's no longer medically necessary, it should be removed promptly.

Use Chlorhexidine Baths: For intensive care patients, daily baths with chlorhexidine gluconate (CHG) wipes can reduce the risk of CLABSIs.

Limit Line Access: Every time the central line is accessed, there's a risk of introducing pathogens. Minimize this by reducing unnecessary checks or medication administrations via the central line.

Adopt Needleless Connectors: Use needleless connectors to reduce the risk of contamination during connection and disconnection procedures. Ensure staff is trained in the proper cleaning of these connectors.

Stay Updated on Technology and Best Practices: As technology evolves, new devices, techniques, and materials might emerge that can reduce CLABSI risks. Stay informed and be ready to adapt.

CLABSIs, though daunting, are largely preventable with vigilant care, stringent protocols, and ongoing education. The gravity of their potential consequences mandates an unwavering commitment to prevention. It's crucial to remember that every central line insertion or maintenance procedure offers both a challenge and an opportunity. By consistently adopting and promoting best practices, healthcare professionals can not only prevent these infections but also champion a culture of patient safety and excellence in care. Every patient, every line, every day—attention to detail can make all the difference.

Ventilator-Associated Pneumonia (VAP)

Ventilator-associated pneumonia (VAP) stands out as a severe and frequent complication in patients requiring mechanical ventilation. VAP, as the term implies, is a type of lung infection (pneumonia) that develops in patients who are on ventilators. Addressing this condition is critical, as it can significantly impact patient outcomes, prolonging hospital stays and increasing medical costs.

Understanding VAP: VAP is an inflammation of the lung caused by infectious agents, specifically occurring more than 48 hours after a patient has been intubated and received mechanical ventilation. Because the ventilator bypasses many of the body's natural defenses against infections, the risk of pneumonia becomes elevated.

Symptoms of VAP: Common manifestations of VAP include:

- Fever or unusually low body temperature.
- New or worsening cough.
- Purulent (pus-like) or increased secretions from the airways.
- Shortness of breath or increased respiratory rate.
- Changes in oxygenation levels.
- Abnormal lung sounds upon examination.
- Radiological evidence showing new or progressive infiltrate.

Factors Contributing to VAP: Several factors can increase the risk of a patient developing VAP:

- **Duration of Ventilation:** The longer a patient remains on a ventilator, the higher the risk.
- **Patient's Overall Health:** Patients with compromised immune systems are more susceptible.
- **Aspiration:** Inhalation of secretions or stomach contents into the lungs can introduce pathogens.
- **Cross-contamination:** This can arise from contaminated equipment or hands.

Tips to Avoid VAP

Elevate the Head of the Bed: Keep patients in a semi-recumbent position, elevating the head of the bed between 30 to 45 degrees unless contraindicated. This reduces the risk of aspiration.

Oral Care: Regularly clean the patient's mouth with antiseptic solutions, like chlorhexidine gluconate. This can reduce the number of pathogens in the mouth that could be aspirated.

Daily "Sedation Vacations": Regularly assess the patient's need for sedation and, when appropriate, reduce sedative medications to assess if the patient can breathe without the ventilator. This can lead to earlier removal from the ventilator.

Assess Daily the Need for Mechanical Ventilation: Evaluate patients daily to determine if they can be safely extubated, thus reducing the time they spend on the ventilator.

Use of Endotracheal Tubes with Subglottic Suctioning: These special tubes allow secretions that collect above the cuff of the endotracheal tube to be aspirated, reducing the risk of them being inhaled into the lungs.

Hand Hygiene: It can't be stressed enough: healthcare providers must regularly and thoroughly wash their hands, especially before and after contact with the patient or the ventilator.

Regular Maintenance and Cleaning of Ventilators: Ensure that all components of the ventilator system are adequately cleaned and maintained to reduce the risk of bacterial colonization.

Limit Transfers and Transport: Whenever possible, limit transporting the patient out of the ICU. If transport is necessary, take precautions to minimize the risk of infections.

Avoid Pooling of Secretions: Regularly check and drain any condensation that forms in the ventilator tubing. This prevents the pooling of secretions, which can be a source of infection.

Stay Updated: Healthcare workers should be routinely trained on the latest guidelines and research related to VAP prevention. Regular audits and feedback mechanisms can also help in maintaining the best practices.

Preventing Ventilator-Associated Pneumonia is a responsibility shared by all members of the healthcare team. By implementing and strictly adhering to evidence-based protocols, it's possible to significantly reduce the incidence of VAP, ensuring that patients receive the safest, highest-quality care. While the mechanics of ventilation might be complex, the steps to prevent VAP are grounded in basic principles of hygiene, patient assessment, and diligent monitoring. As healthcare professionals, every interaction with a ventilated patient presents an opportunity to combat VAP, an endeavor that can save lives and improve overall outcomes.

Clostridium difficile Infections

Clostridium difficile, often referred to as C. diff, is a bacterium that can cause symptoms ranging from diarrhea to life-threatening inflammation of the colon. Of particular concern in healthcare settings, C. difficile infections (CDIs) are notorious for their recurrence and the challenges they pose in treatment and prevention.

Understanding C. difficile: C. difficile is a spore-forming, gram-positive anaerobic bacterium. It becomes problematic primarily in situations where the natural gut flora is disturbed, often due to antibiotic use. When these beneficial bacteria are reduced, C. difficile can thrive and produce toxins that harm the lining of the intestines, leading to CDI symptoms.

Symptoms of CDIs: Manifestations of a C. difficile infection can range from mild to severe and include:
- Watery diarrhea occurs at least three times a day for two or more days.
- Mild abdominal cramping and tenderness.
- Severe abdominal pain.
- Fever.
- Blood or pus in the stool.
- Nausea.
- Dehydration.
- Loss of appetite and weight loss.

In severe cases, it can lead to colon inflammation (colitis), sepsis, and even death.

Factors Contributing to CDIs: While anyone can get a C. difficile infection, certain factors elevate the risk:
- **Antibiotic Use:** Almost any antibiotic can lead to CDI, but broad-spectrum antibiotics pose an exceptionally high risk.
- **Extended Hospital Stays:** The longer one stays in a healthcare setting, the greater the exposure risk.
- **Age:** Older adults, especially those above 65, are at higher risk.
- **Weakened Immune System:** Conditions or medications that suppress the immune system can increase vulnerability.
- **Previous CDI:** Once you've had a C. difficile infection, you're at a higher risk of recurrence.

Tips to Avoid CDIs

Judicious Use of Antibiotics: Only use antibiotics when necessary and precisely as prescribed. Avoid unnecessary use of broad-spectrum antibiotics.

Hand Hygiene: Washing hands with soap and water is the gold standard, especially after using the restroom and before eating. C. diff spores are resistant to alcohol-based hand sanitizers, so handwashing is more effective in this context.

Use Personal Protective Equipment (PPE): Healthcare workers should wear gloves and gowns when treating patients with CDIs. This PPE should be removed and discarded before leaving the patient's room.

Environmental Cleaning: Regularly clean and disinfect surfaces, especially in healthcare settings. Because C. diff spores can survive on surfaces for weeks or even months, it's vital to use products effective against C. diff, like bleach-based cleaners.

Isolate Infected Patients: To prevent the spread in healthcare facilities, patients with CDI should ideally have a private room or share a room only with someone with the same infection.

Educate Healthcare Workers: Continuous training about CDI risks, symptoms, and prevention strategies is crucial.

Monitor Antibiotic Prescribing: Implement antibiotic stewardship programs in healthcare settings to ensure antibiotics are used only when beneficial and necessary.

Prompt Diagnosis and Treatment: Early detection and appropriate treatment can reduce the severity of the infection and its spread.

Probiotics: While research is ongoing, some studies suggest certain probiotics can be beneficial when taking antibiotics, potentially reducing the risk of CDIs.

Stay Updated: Healthcare professionals should be aware of the latest guidelines, research, and recommendations related to C. difficile.

C. difficile infections present a significant challenge, particularly in healthcare environments. However, with informed strategies and vigilant prevention practices, their incidence can be reduced. As the adage goes, prevention is better than cure. By prioritizing patient safety, advocating for antibiotic stewardship, and promoting rigorous hygiene standards, healthcare professionals can play a pivotal role in combating the menace of CDIs, ensuring that patient outcomes are optimized, and hospital environments remain safe.

QUESTIONS AND ANSWERS

Q: What ethical considerations should a CNA consider when caring for a dying person?
A: CNAs should respect the autonomy and wishes of the dying person, including their decisions about life-sustaining treatments and end-of-life care. They must maintain confidentiality, provide honest and accurate information, and avoid imposing their personal beliefs on the patient. It's also important to recognize and address any ethical dilemmas by consulting with the nursing staff and following the healthcare facility's policies.

Q: How should a CNA manage symptoms of anxiety or agitation in a dying person?
A: Managing anxiety or agitation involves creating a calm and soothing environment, using gentle reassurance, and engaging in calming activities like reading or playing soft music. CNAs should report these symptoms to the nursing staff, as they may indicate underlying issues that require medical intervention.

Q: What are the best practices for a CNA when providing hygiene care to a dying person?
A: Best practices include being gentle, respecting the person's privacy and dignity, and being attentive to their comfort and pain levels. It's essential to use a soft touch, avoid causing pain or discomfort, and adjust the care to the person's tolerance. Regular mouth care, keeping the skin clean and dry, and changing positions to avoid bedsores are also crucial.

Q: How can a CNA help manage shortness of breath in a dying patient?
A: CNAs can assist by ensuring the patient is comfortable, such as sitting up or with the head of the bed elevated, providing a fan or cool air for comfort, and ensuring the room has good airflow. They should also promptly report this symptom to the nursing staff for further assessment and management.

Q: What is the significance of advanced directives, and how do they impact CNA care?
A: Advanced directives are legal documents that outline a person's preferences for end-of-life care and medical treatments. They are significant as they guide healthcare providers in making decisions that align with patients' wishes. CNAs must be aware of these directives and ensure the care provided is consistent with the patient's stated preferences.

Q: How should a CNA respect patient autonomy?
A: Respecting patient autonomy is a fundamental ethical principle in healthcare. It involves acknowledging patients' right to make informed decisions about their care and treatment. CNAs demonstrate respect for independence by providing patients with the necessary information, respecting their choices and preferences, and supporting their decision-making ability. For instance, if a patient chooses not to participate in a particular treatment or activity, the CNA should respect this decision, ensure the patient understands the consequences, and report the decision to the supervising nurse.

Q: What is the CNA's responsibility in end-of-life care?
A: In end-of-life care, CNAs are crucial in providing compassionate support to patients and their families. They focus on comfort measures, such as ensuring the patient is pain-free, clean, and comfortable. CNAs also provide emotional support, listening to and acknowledging patients' and their families' feelings and concerns. They must respect the patients' and families' wishes regarding care and treatment and promptly communicate any patient condition changes to the nursing staff.

Q: How should a CNA approach cultural sensitivity in care?
A: Cultural sensitivity is critical to providing effective and respectful patient care. CNAs should recognize and respect cultural differences affecting care practices, communication, dietary preferences, and religious beliefs. This might involve asking patients about their cultural needs, adapting care practices to accommodate cultural norms, and being mindful of cultural differences in body language and communication styles. Understanding and respecting these differences can enhance patient comfort, improve communication, and foster a respectful caregiving environment.

Q: What is palliative care, and how is it relevant to the care of a dying person?
A: Palliative care is a type of care focused on relieving the symptoms and stress of a severe illness. Its goal is to improve the patients' and families' quality of life. For a dying person, palliative care involves managing symptoms such as pain, nausea, and breathlessness and providing psychological, social, and spiritual support. CNAs play a crucial role in palliative care by assisting with daily activities, providing emotional support, and communicating changes in patients' condition to nurses and doctors.

Q: What are the signs of approaching death should CNAs be aware of?
A: CNAs should be aware of several signs that may indicate death is approaching, including increased restlessness, confusion or withdrawal, changes in breathing patterns, decreased intake of food and fluids, and changes in skin color or temperature. Recognizing these signs is essential for providing appropriate care and communicating with the care team and family members.

Q: How can a CNA effectively communicate with a dying person?
A: Effective communication with a dying person includes being present, listening actively, and showing empathy. CNAs should use clear, simple language and be sensitive to the patient's emotional state. Recognizing non-verbal cues is essential, as the person may have difficulty speaking. Providing reassurance and comfort through words and actions is critical.

Q: What is the importance of maintaining a patient's dignity at the end of life?
A: Maintaining a patient's dignity at the end of life is crucial for their emotional and psychological well-being. This includes respecting their privacy, understanding their preferences and values, and involving them in decision-making as much as possible. CNAs contribute by providing respectful and compassionate care, ensuring the patient's comfort, and honoring their wishes.

Q: How should a CNA approach pain management for a dying person?
A: Pain management is a critical aspect of end-of-life care. CNAs should regularly monitor the patient for signs of pain, understanding that they might be non-verbal. They should report any symptoms of pain to the nursing staff promptly. Additionally, CNAs can help by ensuring the patient is comfortable, using pillows for support, and providing non-pharmacological interventions like massage or relaxation techniques, as appropriate.

Q: What role does a CNA play in supporting the family of a dying person?
A: CNAs support the family by providing information about the patient's condition and care, offering emotional support, and guiding them to interact with and care for the dying person. They can also provide practical assistance and information about grief and bereavement support resources.

Q: How can a CNA assist with the spiritual needs of a dying person?
A: CNAs can assist with spiritual needs by facilitating access to spiritual care resources, such as contacting a chaplain or spiritual advisor if requested. They should also respect the patient's religious beliefs and practices and provide a peaceful and respectful environment for any spiritual or religious rituals the patient or family wishes to perform.

Q: How can a CNA support a patient experiencing difficulty eating or drinking?
A: CNAs can support patients by offering small, frequent meals or snacks, assisting with feeding if needed, and providing comfortable, upright positions during meal times. They should also monitor for discomfort or difficulty swallowing and report these to the nursing staff.

Q: What should a CNA consider when managing incontinence in a dying patient?
A: Managing incontinence involves regular checking and changing to keep the patient clean and comfortable, using absorbent pads or briefs as needed, and being sensitive to the patient's dignity and privacy. Good skin care is also essential to prevent irritation and sores.

Q: How can a CNA identify and support a patient experiencing delirium or confusion at the end of life?
A: CNAs can identify delirium or confusion by noting changes in the patient's level of consciousness, attention, thinking, and perception. Providing a calm, reassuring presence, speaking in a soft, clear voice, and maintaining a quiet, well-lit environment can help. Reporting these changes to the nursing staff for further assessment is essential.

Q: What role does a CNA play in grief and bereavement support for families?
A: CNAs support grieving families by offering compassionate listening, providing information about grief resources, and being present and available to assist with immediate needs. They can also share memories of the patient and acknowledge the family's loss, showing respect and empathy.

Q: How should a CNA address a patient's fears or concerns about dying?
A: Addressing fears and concerns involves listening empathetically, reassuring, and respecting the patient's feelings. CNAs should encourage the expression of feelings and, if appropriate, facilitate conversations with family members or the healthcare team about these concerns.

Q: What are the guidelines for a CNA when handling medications for a dying person?
A: CNAs should follow strict guidelines for medication handling, including verifying the medication, dosage, and timing as prescribed and observing the patient for any adverse reactions or side effects. They should also document medication administration accurately and report any concerns to the nursing staff.

Q: How can a CNA create a peaceful environment for dying people?
A: Creating a peaceful environment involves maintaining a quiet, calm atmosphere, managing light and noise levels, and personalizing the space with items comforting to the patient, such as photos or soft music. Respecting the patient's need for privacy and rest periods is also essential.

Q: What strategies can CNAs use to cope with their own emotions when caring for a dying person?
A: CNAs can cope with their emotions by seeking colleague support, participating in debriefing sessions, utilizing employee assistance programs, and practicing self-care activities such as exercise, hobbies, or relaxation techniques. Acknowledging and expressing emotions healthily is critical to managing the emotional impact of this work.

Q: How can a CNA assist with post-mortem care?
A: Post-mortem care involves cleaning and preparing the body according to facility policies and the family's wishes, ensuring dignity and respect for the deceased. CNAs should also assist with the logistical aspects of post-mortem care, such as coordinating with the funeral home and supporting the family as needed.

Q: What is the role of a CNA in documenting care for a dying person?
A: CNA documentation is crucial for maintaining accurate records of the care provided, including changes in the patient's condition, symptoms, and intervention responses. This documentation aids communication among the care team and ensures continuity of care.

Q: What are the critical steps in performing proper hand hygiene?
A: Proper hand hygiene includes wetting hands with water, applying soap, rubbing hands together for at least 20 seconds, covering all surfaces, rinsing thoroughly under running water, and drying with a disposable towel. This process is crucial in preventing the spread of infections.

Q: What is patient confidentiality and its importance for a CNA?
A: Patient confidentiality refers to the ethical and legal duty of CNAs to keep all information about patients private. This includes personal details, medical history, and treatment plans. CNAS must adhere to these standards to respect patient privacy, build trust, and comply with legal requirements like the Health Insurance Portability and Accountability Act (HIPAA). Breaches of confidentiality can lead to legal consequences, damage the trust between patient and caregiver, and compromise the integrity of the healthcare facility.

Q: How should a CNA handle a situation where a patient refuses care?
A: When a patient refuses care, a CNA must respect the patient's autonomy and decision. They should ensure the patient is informed about the implications of refusing care. The refusal and information provided to the patient should be documented accurately in the patient's record. It's also crucial to report the refusal to a supervising nurse or doctor, as they may need to assess the patient's capacity to make decisions or provide additional information that might change the patient's decision. This respect for patient choice is a fundamental ethical principle in healthcare.

Q: What is informed consent, and does a CNA handle it?

A: Informed consent is when a patient is provided with information about a medical procedure or treatment, including its risks, benefits, and alternatives, and then consents to receive it. While CNAs are not typically responsible for obtaining informed consent, they play a supportive role. This can involve relaying patients' questions to nurses or doctors, helping patients understand the information, and observing any concerns or hesitations that patients might express about the treatment. CNAs should be aware of the informed consent process as it ensures that patient care is based on an understanding and agreement.

Q: Can a CNA accept gifts from patients?

A: Accepting gifts from patients can be a complex issue for CNAs. While small tokens of appreciation might be acceptable, accepting donations of significant value can create ethical dilemmas and potential conflicts of interest. It might be perceived as favoritism or influence the care provided. CNAs should adhere to the policies of their employing facility regarding gifts and generally err on the side of caution. If offered assistance, it's often best to politely decline or discuss the situation with a supervisor to ensure that professional boundaries are maintained and ethical standards are upheld.

Q: What is the role of a CNA in maintaining patient dignity?

A: Maintaining patient dignity is fundamental to a CNA's role. This involves treating each patient respectfully and kindly, regardless of their condition or background. It includes practical steps like ensuring privacy during personal care tasks, such as bathing and toileting, listening to and honoring their preferences in daily care, and using a respectful tone of voice. For instance, when assisting with personal hygiene, a CNA should use draping techniques to expose only the necessary areas of the patient's body. These actions demonstrate respect for the patient and help preserve their sense of self-worth and dignity.

Q: How should a CNA respond to suspected abuse or neglect?

A: If a CNA suspects abuse or neglect, they have a legal and ethical obligation to report it immediately to a supervisor or the appropriate authorities in the facility. This could include signs of physical, emotional, or financial abuse or neglect of a patient's basic needs. The CNA should document their observations clearly and factually without making assumptions about the cause. Timely reporting is crucial as it can trigger an investigation and ensure the safety and well-being of the patient. CNAs must be aware that failure to report suspected abuse or neglect can have profound legal implications and go against the ethical standards of patient care.

Q: What is a CNA's responsibility in documentation?

A: Accurate and honest documentation by CNAs is vital for effective patient care and legal compliance. CNAs must record relevant patient information, such as vital signs, intake and output, and any patient condition changes. Documentation should be timely, clear, and factual, avoiding subjective interpretations. It is a critical communication tool among the healthcare team and is essential for continuity of care. Furthermore, in legal terms, accurate documentation can provide evidence of care and protect the CNA and healthcare facility in litigation cases.

Q: How can CNAs ensure they practice within their scope of work?

A: CNAs should be thoroughly familiar with the scope of practice defined by their state's regulations and the policies of their employing healthcare facility. This includes understanding the tasks they are legally permitted to perform and recognizing those that require higher-level professional skills, such as administering medication or performing invasive procedures. CNAs should communicate this to their supervisor and request guidance or additional training if asked to complete a task outside their scope. Staying within the range of practice is crucial for patient safety and professional integrity.

Q: What is the importance of ethical behavior in CNA practice?

A: Ethical behavior is foundational to the CNA's role in healthcare. It encompasses principles such as respect for patients, honesty, compassion, and responsibility. Ethical CNAs build trust with patients and colleagues, contributing to a positive healthcare environment. They make decisions that prioritize patient well-being, respect patient rights, and comply with legal and professional standards. Ethical conduct also includes reporting unethical behavior observed in the workplace, which upholds the nursing profession's standards and ensures high-quality patient care.

Q: How should a CNA manage personal health information?
A: CNAs must handle personal health information with confidentiality and security. This includes discussing patient information only with authorized personnel involved in the patient's care and avoiding conversations about patients in public areas where they can be overheard. CNAs must also be cautious with written and electronic records, ensuring they are accessible only to authorized individuals. Compliance with HIPAA and other privacy laws is essential in protecting patient information from unauthorized access or disclosure, which can lead to legal repercussions and damage to the healthcare facility's reputation.

Q: What should a CNA do if they make a medication error?
A: In a medication error, immediate and transparent action is required. The CNA should promptly report the error to a supervising nurse or physician, regardless of whether the mistake seems minor or if the patient appears unharmed. Early reporting allows for timely intervention to mitigate potential harm to the patient. The CNA should also document the incident accurately in the patient's record. This honesty in reporting is crucial for patient safety, enables the healthcare team to learn from mistakes, and is a fundamental aspect of professional accountability.

Q: Can a CNA witness legal documents for patients?
A: CNAs are generally not authorized to witness legal documents for patients, such as advance directives or wills. This role is typically reserved for notaries, the public, lawyers, or other legally authorized individuals. CNAs should focus on their primary patient care responsibilities and leave legal matters to appropriately authorized personnel. If a patient requests assistance with legal documents, the CNA should refer the matter to a supervisor or the appropriate department within the facility.

Q: What is a CNA's role in advance directives?
A: CNAs should know a patient's advance directives, such as living wills or durable power of attorney for healthcare. These documents express the patient's medical treatment preferences, especially when they cannot make decisions themselves. While CNAs do not play a role in creating or executing these directives, they must ensure that the care provided aligns with the stipulations outlined in them. This may involve communicating the existence of these directives to nurses and other team members involved in the patient's care.

Q: How should a CNA assist a patient with brushing their teeth?
A: Assist the patient by preparing the toothbrush with toothpaste. Support the patient in brushing all surfaces of their teeth. If the patient cannot spit, use a swab to clean the mouth. Always be gentle and respectful of the patient's comfort and preferences.

Q: What are the guidelines for bathing a patient in bed?
A: Ensure privacy, explain the procedure, check water temperature, and start from the cleanest to the least clean areas. Use a gentle soap, rinse, and dry each room thoroughly. Regularly check for any skin changes or pressure sores.

Q: Describe how to make an occupied bed properly.
A: Ensure the patient's safety and comfort. Loosen the bed linen, then replace the bottom sheet, starting from the side furthest from you. Roll the patient gently onto the clean linen, then do the same on the other side. Change pillowcases and top sheets while minimizing discomfort to the patient.

Q: What is the correct procedure for dressing a patient with a weak right arm?
A: Start by dressing the weaker right arm first. Gently guide the arm through the sleeve, then dress the more muscular left arm. Ensure the clothing is comfortable and ask for the patient's preference throughout the process.

Q: How do you safely transfer a patient from a bed to a wheelchair?
A: Use a gait belt for support, and ensure the wheelchair is locked and close to the bed. Assist the patient to sit, stand, and pivot towards the wheelchair. Gently lower them into the wheelchair, ensuring they are comfortable and secure.

Q: What are the essential considerations when providing nail care?
A: Check the patient's hands and feet for cuts, sores, or nail conditions. Soak the nails, trim them straight across, and gently smooth any rough edges. Be cautious not to cut too close to the skin.

Q: How should a CNA assist with toileting using a bedpan?
A: Explain the procedure, provide privacy, and position the bedpan correctly under the patient. After use, assist the patient off the bedpan, clean and dry the perineal area, and ensure comfort and hygiene.

Q: Describe the procedure for measuring a patient's urinary output.
A: Use a graduated container to measure the urine. Record the amount accurately in milliliters, observe the color and clarity, and report any unusual findings to the nurse. Ensure proper disposal and hygiene practices.

Q: What is the importance of oral hygiene for unconscious patients?
A: Regular oral hygiene prevents infection and keeps the mouth moist. Use a swab to clean the teeth, gums, and tongue gently. Avoid toothpaste and ensure the head is turned to the side to prevent aspiration.

Q: How do you assist a patient with shaving?
A: Ensure the patient's consent, use either an electric or safety razor, apply shaving cream, and shave in the direction of hair growth. Be extra careful to avoid cuts, especially in patients with blood thinners.

Q: Explain how to provide perineal care for a female patient.
A: Explain the procedure, provide privacy, and use warm water and mild soap. Clean from front to back, rinse and dry thoroughly. Always be gentle and respectful, ensuring the patient's comfort.

Q: What are the steps in foot care for a diabetic patient?
A: Inspect the feet for any sores or abnormalities, wash with lukewarm water and mild soap, dry thoroughly, especially between the toes, apply moisturizer but not between toes, and avoid cutting nails without specific instructions.

Q: How should a CNA position a patient to prevent pressure ulcers?
A: Regularly change the patient's position at least every two hours, use pillows for support, check skin integrity, and ensure the bedding is smooth and wrinkle-free.

Q: What are the common signs and symptoms of dehydration in elderly patients?
A: Common signs of dehydration in elderly patients include dry mouth, sunken eyes, dark yellow urine, dry skin, confusion, dizziness, and low blood pressure. CNAS needs to monitor patients closely, encourage fluid intake, and promptly report concerning symptoms to the nursing staff due to the severe consequences of dehydration, such as exacerbating other health issues.

Q: How can a CNA assist arthritis patients in their daily activities?
A: CNAs can support arthritis patients by conducting gentle joint mobility exercises to maintain or improve joint flexibility. They can also help with activities of daily living (ADLs), administer prescribed pain medications, ensure a comfortable and accessible living environment, and offer emotional support to help patients cope with the challenges of chronic pain.

Q: What are pressure ulcers, and how can CNAs help prevent them?
A: Pressure ulcers, or bedsores, result from prolonged pressure on specific body areas, primarily in bedridden or immobile patients. CNAs play a crucial role in prevention by repositioning patients regularly, maintaining proper skin hygiene, using pressure-relieving devices, ensuring adequate nutrition, and promptly reporting any concerning skin changes to the healthcare team.

Q: Describe the emotional impact of a sudden illness diagnosis on a patient.
A: A sudden illness diagnosis can evoke various emotional responses in patients, including shock, fear, anxiety, depression, and denial. CNAs should offer empathetic emotional support, encourage open communication, and involve the healthcare team in addressing these complex emotions to help patients cope effectively.

Q: How can CNAs assist patients with chronic pain management?

A: CNAs can support patients with chronic pain by monitoring and documenting pain levels, administering prescribed pain medications, assisting with relaxation techniques, and promoting activities that provide distraction from pain, such as music therapy or engaging in hobbies.

Q: What is the role of CNAs in managing patients with dementia?

A: CNAs are crucial in providing a safe and supportive environment for dementia patients. Their responsibilities include using gentle redirection to manage behavior, maintaining consistent routines, offering emotional support, and promptly reporting any changes in behavior to the nursing team.

Q: How can CNAs promote mobility and prevent muscle atrophy in bedridden patients?

A: CNAs can promote mobility in bedridden patients by performing passive range of motion exercises, assisting with transfers, utilizing assistive devices like walkers or canes, and encouraging regular position changes to prevent muscle atrophy and maintain joint flexibility.

Q: Explain the importance of maintaining good oral hygiene in elderly patients.

A: Good oral hygiene is essential for preventing dental issues, pneumonia, and malnutrition in elderly patients. CNAs should assist with daily oral care, monitor for oral problems, and encourage regular dental check-ups to ensure the overall well-being of their patients.

Q: What are the common signs of depression in elderly patients, and how can CNAs provide emotional support?

A: Signs of depression in elderly patients may include social withdrawal, changes in appetite, sleep disturbances, and persistent feelings of sadness. CNAs can provide emotional support by actively listening, engaging in conversation, encouraging participation in activities, and promptly reporting concerns to the healthcare team for further evaluation and intervention.

Q: How can CNAs help patients with respiratory conditions, such as COPD, manage their symptoms?

A: CNAs can assist patients with respiratory conditions by ensuring a clean and clutter-free environment, monitoring oxygen levels, helping with prescribed respiratory treatments, encouraging proper breathing techniques, and recognizing and promptly reporting any signs of respiratory distress, such as increased shortness of breath or cyanosis.

Q: What are the critical considerations for CNAs when caring for patients with diabetes?

A: When caring for diabetic patients, CNAs should monitor blood glucose levels, assist with insulin administration or glucose monitoring, promote a balanced diet, encourage regular exercise, and be vigilant for signs of hypo or hyperglycemia. They should also support diabetic patients adhering to their prescribed treatment plans and report any concerning symptoms to the nursing staff.

Q: How can CNAs assist patients who are recovering from surgery?

A: CNAs can support post-surgery patients by monitoring vital signs, assisting with wound care and dressing changes, administering prescribed medications, assisting with mobility and ambulation, ensuring patients adhere to dietary restrictions, and providing emotional support during the recovery process.

Q: Explain the importance of infection control in healthcare settings and how CNAs can contribute to it.

A: Infection control is crucial for preventing the spread of infectious diseases in healthcare settings. CNAs can contribute by practicing proper hand hygiene, using personal protective equipment (PPE), following isolation precautions when necessary, disinfecting equipment and surfaces, and educating patients and their families about infection prevention measures to maintain a safe and sterile environment.

Q: What is the role of CNAs in end-of-life care?

A: In end-of-life care, CNAs play a compassionate role by providing comfort measures, assisting with personal care and pain management, facilitating communication between patients and their families, and ensuring patients' dignity and comfort during their final moments.

Q: How can CNAs recognize and respond to elder abuse or neglect signs?
A: CNAs should be vigilant for signs of elder abuse or neglect, such as unexplained injuries, changes in behavior, malnutrition, or dehydration. If they suspect abuse or neglect, they must report it to their supervisor or appropriate authorities to ensure the safety and well-being of the elderly patient.

Q: Describe the importance of maintaining patient confidentiality and privacy in healthcare.
A: Maintaining patient confidentiality and privacy is critical to building trust and ensuring ethical care. CNAs must safeguard patient information, follow HIPAA regulations, and conduct conversations and care activities discreetly to protect patients' dignity and sensitive medical information.

Q: How can CNAs assist patients with visual or hearing impairments daily?
A: CNAs can support patients with visual impairments by providing verbal cues, offering assistance with mobility, ensuring a clutter-free environment, and facilitating communication through tactile or auditory methods. For patients with hearing impairments, using clear and straightforward communication, employing gestures or sign language if necessary, and ensuring hearing aids function properly are essential steps for adequate care.

Q: What is the role of CNAs in preventing falls among elderly patients?
A: CNAs play a crucial role in fall prevention by conducting fall risk assessments, ensuring the environment is free of hazards, assisting with mobility and transfers, and using assistive devices like walkers or handrails as needed. They should also educate patients and families about fall prevention strategies.

Q: How can CNAs help patients with anxiety disorders manage their symptoms?
A: CNAs can support patients with anxiety disorders by providing a calm and reassuring presence, promoting relaxation techniques like deep breathing exercises, assisting with prescribed medications, and facilitating a structured routine to reduce stress and anxiety triggers.

Q: Explain the importance of maintaining a patient's dignity and respecting their cultural beliefs and preferences.
A: Maintaining a patient's dignity and respecting their cultural beliefs and preferences are fundamental principles of patient-centered care. CNAs should address patients respectfully, use appropriate terminology, honor cultural traditions, and provide care that aligns with the patient's values and preferences to ensure their emotional and psychological well-being.

Q: How can CNAs assist patients with cognitive impairments, such as Alzheimer's disease, in their daily activities?
A: CNAs can support patients with cognitive impairments by establishing a routine, using simple and clear communication, offering reminders for daily tasks, ensuring a safe environment, and engaging in meaningful activities that promote cognitive stimulation and social interaction.

Q: What is the role of CNAs in promoting a positive patient experience and satisfaction?
A: CNAs contribute to a positive patient experience by providing compassionate care, actively listening to patients' needs and concerns, maintaining open communication, ensuring comfort and safety, and promptly addressing any issues or requests to enhance patient satisfaction and well-being.

Q: How does the approach to care differ when caring for pediatric patients compared to elderly patients?
A: The approach to care varies based on age. With pediatric patients, a gentle and child-friendly approach, focusing on communication with the child and their parents, is essential. Elderly patients require patience and respect for their independence while addressing age-related health concerns.

Q: What are some common age-related changes in the elderly population that CNAs should be aware of?
A: Age-related changes in the elderly may include reduced mobility, sensory impairments (vision and hearing), cognitive decline, and increased susceptibility to chronic diseases. CNAs should tailor care to accommodate these changes.

Q: How can CNAs support family members when caring for patients at the end of life?
A: CNAs can provide emotional support to family members by listening to their concerns, offering information about the patient's condition, facilitating communication with the healthcare team, and helping create a comfortable and peaceful environment for the patient and their family.

Q: Describe the importance of maintaining a patient's dignity when caring for all age groups.
A: Maintaining patient dignity is vital in all age groups. CNAs should respect patients' privacy, use appropriate communication, and ensure their comfort, regardless of age, to preserve their self-worth and respect.

Q: How can CNAs assist in providing culturally competent care for patients from diverse backgrounds?
A: CNAs should respect cultural beliefs, practices, and preferences. They can seek guidance from patients and their families, engage in cultural competency training, and collaborate with interpreters when necessary to ensure patients receive culturally sensitive care.

Q: What are some fundamental principles of infection control in healthcare settings?
A: Key principles of infection control include proper hand hygiene, personal protective equipment (PPE) use, adherence to isolation precautions, regular disinfection of equipment and surfaces, and education of patients and staff on infection prevention.

Q: How can CNAs contribute to preventing hospital-acquired infections (HAIs)?
A: CNAs play a role in HAI prevention by practicing good hand hygiene, using PPE when required, ensuring clean patient environments, and promoting infection control measures among patients and healthcare staff.

Q: What are the benefits of early detection and management of chronic diseases?
A: Early detection and management of chronic diseases can lead to better health outcomes, improved quality of life, and reduced healthcare costs. CNAs should assist in monitoring patients' chronic conditions and adherence to treatment plans.

Q: How can CNAs support patients in maintaining a healthy lifestyle?
A: CNAs can encourage and educate patients on adopting a healthy lifestyle by promoting regular exercise, balanced nutrition, smoking cessation, and stress management techniques. They can also assist in adhering to prescribed health regimens.

Q: Describe the role of CNAs in promoting medication safety among patients.
A: CNAs can contribute to medication safety by administering medications accurately, documenting administration, monitoring for side effects, and educating patients on proper medication use. They should report any medication errors or concerns promptly.

Q: What measures can CNAs take to prevent patient falls in healthcare settings?
A: To prevent patient falls, CNAs should perform fall risk assessments, keep the environment free of hazards, assist with mobility, use assistive devices as needed, and educate patients about fall prevention techniques.

Q: How can CNAs assist patients in managing and adhering to their prescribed treatment plans?
A: CNAs can support patients by providing clear instructions, offering reminders for medications and appointments, monitoring progress, and reporting any concerns or non-adherence issues to the healthcare team.

Q: Explain the importance of maintaining patient confidentiality and privacy in healthcare.
A: Maintaining patient confidentiality and privacy is essential to build trust and protect sensitive medical information. CNAs must adhere to HIPAA regulations, ensure discreet communication, and safeguard patient records.

Q: What strategies can CNAs employ to promote a positive patient experience and satisfaction?
A: CNAs can promote a positive patient experience by providing compassionate care, actively listening to patients' needs and concerns, maintaining open communication, ensuring comfort and safety, and promptly addressing any issues or requests to enhance patient satisfaction and well-being.

Q: How can CNAs assist in preventing readmissions to healthcare facilities?
A: CNAs can help prevent readmissions by ensuring patients understand their discharge instructions, providing education on managing their conditions at home, assisting with medication management, and promoting follow-up appointments with healthcare providers.

Q: What everyday health promotion activities can CNAs engage in with patients?
A: CNAs can engage in health promotion activities like educating patients on healthy eating habits, encouraging regular exercise, supporting smoking cessation efforts, providing information on immunizations, and promoting stress reduction techniques.

Q: What is the role of CNAs in disaster preparedness and response within healthcare facilities?
A: CNAs play a crucial role in disaster preparedness by assisting in developing emergency plans, conducting drills, and ensuring patient safety during emergencies. They also provide care to patients during and after disasters. This involves helping to create and implement disaster plans, participating in regular disaster drills, and staying updated on emergency protocols.

Q: How can CNAs assist in evacuating patients during a healthcare facility emergency?
A: CNAs can assist in patient evacuation by following facility evacuation protocols, helping mobilize patients, ensuring patient records and medications are accessible, and providing emotional support during the process. They may also assist with moving patients to designated evacuation areas and helping to ensure a smooth and orderly evacuation process.

Q: What steps should CNAs take to ensure patient safety during a fire emergency?
A: To ensure patient safety during a fire, CNAs should follow facility fire safety protocols, including closing doors, using fire extinguishers if trained, assisting with evacuation, and reporting the fire to appropriate personnel. Additionally, they should remain calm and help keep patients calm during the emergency.

Q: How can CNAs assist in managing patients during a natural disaster, such as a hurricane or flood?
A: CNAs can assist in managing patients during a natural disaster by ensuring patients are safe and dry, helping with moving patients to safer areas, providing emotional support, and reporting any medical issues promptly to the healthcare team. They should also be prepared to adapt to changing conditions and follow disaster protocols.

Q: Explain the importance of having a disaster supply kit in a healthcare facility.
A: A disaster supply kit in a healthcare facility is essential to ensure that necessary supplies, medications, and equipment are readily available during emergencies. CNAs should help maintain and replenish these kits, ensuring that important items like first aid supplies, medications, flashlights, batteries, and communication devices are readily accessible to provide timely care and support during disasters or emergencies.

Q: What actions should CNAs take when encountering a patient with a suspected contagious disease, such as tuberculosis (TB)?
A: When encountering a patient with a suspected contagious disease like tuberculosis, CNAs should follow infection control protocols meticulously. This includes wearing appropriate personal protective equipment (PPE), such as masks and gloves, maintaining proper hand hygiene, educating the patient on respiratory hygiene practices, and promptly reporting the situation to the healthcare team. The goal is to prevent the spread of the contagious disease to other patients and healthcare workers while ensuring the patient receives appropriate care and isolation if necessary.

Q: What measures should CNAs take to ensure patient safety during a power outage in a healthcare facility?
A: CNAs should prioritize patient safety during a power outage in a healthcare facility. They can do so by using flashlights or emergency lighting to provide visibility and emotional support to patients who may be anxious or scared, monitoring patients who rely on life-sustaining equipment to ensure their safety, and promptly reporting any issues or concerns to the healthcare team. It's essential to ensure patients remain comfortable and secure during the outage.

Q: What is the purpose of a disaster drill, and how can CNAs participate effectively?
A: Disaster drills test emergency response plans, prepare healthcare staff for various disaster scenarios, and identify areas for improvement in disaster preparedness and response efforts. CNAs can participate effectively in these drills by actively engaging in the exercises, following established disaster protocols, practicing their specific roles and responsibilities, and providing feedback to help refine and enhance the facility's disaster preparedness efforts. These drills are critical in ensuring that all staff are well-prepared to respond effectively to emergencies.

Q: What steps should CNAs take to maintain their safety during a disaster or emergency?
A: CNAs should prioritize their safety during a disaster or emergency. To do so, they should follow established protocols, use appropriate personal protective equipment (PPE) when necessary, stay informed about the situation and any updates or directives, and evacuate if required while ensuring the patients' safety is crucial for CNAs to balance their dedication to patient care with their well-being to respond to emergencies effectively.

Q: How can CNAs support patients in coping with the emotional aftermath of a disaster or traumatic event?
A: CNAs can provide vital emotional support to patients coping with the aftermath of a disaster or traumatic event. This support includes actively listening to patients, validating their feelings and concerns, offering reassurance, providing information about available resources for counseling or support groups, and helping patients and their families navigate the emotional challenges that may arise. CNAs should be empathetic and understanding, recognizing the psychological impact of such events on individuals and offering a caring presence to assist in the healing process.

Q: What are the critical components of a disaster preparedness plan in a healthcare facility?
A: A disaster preparedness plan in a healthcare facility typically includes several key components. These components may encompass risk assessments to identify potential hazards, emergency communication protocols for staff and patients, evacuation plans, resource allocation strategies to ensure sufficient supplies and personnel, staff training and education, and the implementation of regular disaster drills. The plan aims to provide a structured framework for effectively responding to emergencies and safeguarding the well-being of patients and staff.

Q: How can CNAs assist in caring for vulnerable populations, such as older people or individuals with disabilities, during a disaster?
A: CNAs are critical in providing care to vulnerable populations during disasters. They can ensure the safety of elderly patients or those with disabilities by promptly evacuating them if necessary and assisting with mobility aids or adaptive equipment. CNAs should also provide emotional support to help alleviate the stress and anxiety experienced by these individuals during a crisis. Additionally, they can coordinate care with other healthcare professionals to address the specific needs of vulnerable patients, such as medication management and assistance with daily activities.

Q: Explain the importance of community involvement and collaboration in disaster preparedness and response.
A: Community involvement and collaboration are essential for effective disaster preparedness and response efforts. CNAs should actively participate in community planning initiatives, engage with local authorities and organizations, and build strong partnerships within the community. By doing so, healthcare facilities and CNAs can gain access to valuable resources, share critical information, and coordinate response efforts more effectively when disasters or emergencies occur. Community collaboration enhances the overall response to crises, ensuring a more coordinated and comprehensive approach to safeguarding public health and safety.

Q: What are the potential challenges CNAs may encounter during disaster response, and how can they address them?

A: CNAs may encounter various challenges during disaster response, such as resource shortages, communication barriers, and emotional distress. To address these challenges effectively, CNAs should adapt to changing circumstances, follow established disaster protocols diligently, seek support and guidance from colleagues and supervisors, and engage in self-care practices to manage stress. Open communication with the healthcare team and a willingness to work together can help overcome challenges and ensure a more coordinated and successful response to emergencies.

Q: How can CNAs assist in ensuring the continuity of care for patients with chronic conditions during a disaster?

A: Ensuring the continuity of care for patients with chronic conditions during a disaster is crucial. CNAs can play a vital role by accurately documenting patients' medical histories, treatment plans, and medication regimens. Additionally, they can assist with medication management, ensuring patients have access to necessary medications during the emergency. Effective communication with healthcare providers and emergency responders is essential to address any specific needs or concerns related to chronic conditions and provide uninterrupted care to these patients.

Q: What steps should CNAs take to prepare for a disaster or emergency at work?

A: CNAs should take proactive steps to prepare for a disaster or emergency while at work. This includes familiarizing themselves with the facility's emergency plans and protocols and knowing the location of emergency exits, fire extinguishers, and first aid supplies. CNAs should also actively participate in disaster drills and training sessions to gain confidence in their roles during emergencies. Staying informed about emergency procedures and updates from healthcare leadership is essential to being well-prepared and ready to respond effectively in times of crisis.

Q: How can CNAs assist in maintaining infection control measures during an outbreak or pandemic, such as COVID-19?

A: CNAs can contribute significantly to maintaining infection control measures during an outbreak or pandemic by strictly adhering to infection prevention protocols. This includes practicing proper hand hygiene, wearing appropriate personal protective equipment (PPE), such as masks and gloves, following respiratory hygiene practices, and ensuring proper disinfection of surfaces and equipment. CNAs should also educate patients on preventive measures, such as frequent handwashing and wearing masks when necessary, to reduce the risk of infection transmission. Timely reporting suspected cases or concerns to the healthcare team is essential for early intervention and containment efforts.

CONCLUSION

In conclusion, this practice book was created to give readers a thorough and challenging resource for preparing for the CNA profession. We have covered a wide range of topics, including the duties and roles of a CNA, the critical competencies needed to deliver high-quality patient care, and methods for getting ready for the CNA exam.

To simulate the CNA exam and assist readers in identifying their strengths and shortcomings, we have included a practice test; each question's correct responses come with thorough justifications and annotations on critical ideas.

Additionally, we have offered advice on handling test-day stress, performing better, and sources for further education and CNA career advancement.

We hope this book has been an invaluable resource for people considering a career as a certified nursing assistant and has given readers the information and abilities required to deliver high-quality patient care. Wishing you success as a CNA!

SPECIAL DOWNLOAD

Dear reader, I would be grateful if you would take a minute of your time to share your feedback on the purchase site to let other users know what the experience was like and what you liked best about the book. In addition, I have recently decided to give **extra study aids** to all our readers. Yes, I want to provide you with the assistance that will help you with your study you will receive:

Extra Content 1= **Audiobook**

Extra Content 2= Digital book **"Medical Terminology"**

Extra Content 3= Over **875** Flashcards (pdf and apkg. format *for Anki app or Anki droid*) divided into:

***600 digital flashcards with picture** of general medical terminology

***275 digital flashcards** covering a range of essential topics, including:

- Basic **anatomy** and **physiology** concepts
- Common **diseases** and **conditions**
- Common **medical abbreviations**
- Control and fall **prevention**
- Effective **communication skills** with patients and family
- **Laws** and **regulations** governing the CNA profession
- Pain **management** and wound care techniques
- **Procedures** and **techniques**
- Meal preparation and **nutrition skills**
- Safety **procedures** and **protocols**
- **Vital signs** and how to measure them

Get all flashcards **in PDF and APKG format!** You can track your progress and conveniently and interactively memorize the most important terms and concepts! Download to your device: **Anki APP or AnkiDroid**, or enter the web page and register free of charge. Then import the files we have given you as a gift and use the flashcards whenever and wherever you want to study and track your progress.

Unlock your exclusive study materials!

Simply scan the QR code below to unlock everything instantly.

Need help or have a question?
Write to us at: **info.testbookreader@gmail.com**

Thank you!

Made in United States
Troutdale, OR
05/04/2025

30965260R00044